# APPLIED MEDICAL MICROBIOLOGY

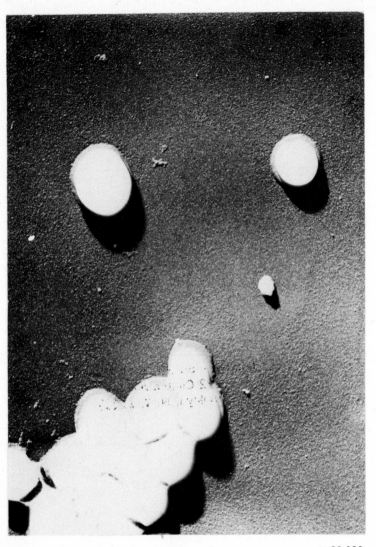

Electron micrograph showing staphylococci.                    × 20 000.

# Basic microbiology

EDITOR: J. F. WILKINSON

# Volume 3

# Applied medical microbiology

## J. G. COLLEE M.D., F.R.C.Path.

Personal Professor of Bacteriology
University Medical School
Edinburgh

A HALSTED PRESS BOOK

JOHN WILEY & SONS

NEW YORK

© 1976 Blackwell Scientific Publications
Osney Mead, Oxford.
85 Marylebone High Street, London, W1M 3DE
9 Forrest Road, Edinburgh,
P.O. Box 9, North Balwyn, Victoria, Australia.

First published 1976


Published in the U.S.A. by
Halsted Press, a Division of
John Wiley & Sons, Inc.,
New York




Library of Congress Cataloging in Publication Data

Collee, J. G.
    Applied medical microbiology

    (Basic microbiology ; v. 3)
    1. Medical Microbiology. I. Title
QR46.C76  1976  616.01  75-42120
ISBN  0-470-15001-7

Printed in Great Britain

# Contents

# Preface

There are several good general textbooks of Medical Microbiology and many specialist texts that deal with aspects of Bacteriology, Virology, Mycology and Protozoology in relation to infectious diseases of man.

This small book cannot bear comparison with any of these volumes. It has been written in the hope that it may set the scene usefully for students of biology, junior medical and dental students, nurses and paraclinical technicians who may seek a gentle introduction to some clinically related areas of microbiology. The aim has been to present concepts and to bring in new facts and terms as they are needed to develop the individual chapters. The use of a limited number of illustrative examples and the repetition of some examples to demonstrate different aspects, or to emphasise important points, is intentional.

It is hoped that, despite the many inadequacies and omissions of this slim volume as a general source of information, it might drive the reader to fuller texts in due course, sufficiently equipped with some of the language and the concepts of Medical Microbiology to tackle the further reading with a measure of understanding and infectious enthusiasm.

I am indebted to many colleagues, particularly to Dr Andrew Fraser, Dr Brian Duerden, Mr William Marr, Dr John Peutherer and Dr Donald Weir, for their constructive advice. I am also grateful to Mr James Paul who did the photomicrography and to Mr Ian Lennox who helped me with some of the original artwork. Special thanks are due to Mr Robert Campbell and his colleagues at Blackwells for their care.

# 1 Introduction

The micro-organisms that abound in Nature are classified on the basis of their size, structure and other criteria, into the groups indicated in Table 1.1 and Fig. 1.1.

**Table 1.1**  Major groups of eukaryotic and prokaryotic organisms and the viruses (a simplified classification).

| | |
|---|---|
| EUKARYOTIC CELLS | Protozoa<br>Algae<br>Fungi (including yeasts) |
| PROKARYOTIC CELLS | Bacteria (including filamentous bacteria)<br>Spirochaetes<br>Rickettsiae<br>Chlamydiae<br>Mycoplasmas |
| . . . | Viruses |

This book deals mainly with the commensal and pathogenic bacteria of man. It includes a brief consideration of some fungi and viruses of medical importance, but it does not deal with pathogenic protozoa.

Micro-organisms that cause disease in plants, animals or Man are called *pathogens* and may be distinguished from the very large group of free-living and generally harmless *saprophytes* that include many organisms involved in natural processes of decomposition and putrefaction. With few exceptions, the pathogens are parasites and cause disease by living on or in a host and interfering in some way with the host metabolism. However, parasitism is not necessarily harmful; there are many micro-organisms that are not free-living but lead a parasitic existence without apparently causing disease in the host. The parasites concerned in this form of peaceful co-existence are known as *commensal organisms.* In some cases, the commensal state is more or less enduring and there are clear examples of symbiosis in which the host-parasite association is mutually beneficial. On the other hand, many commensal organisms may attack the host when special circumstances allow and these organisms are regarded as *potential pathogens.*

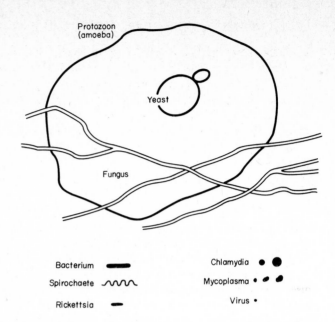

| | | |
|---|---|---|
| Bacterium | ▬ | |
| Spirochaete | ∿∿ | |
| Rickettsia | ▬ | |
| Chlamydia | • ● | |
| Mycoplasma | • ● ● | |
| Virus | • | |

**Figure 1.1** An outline of the relative sizes and approximate shapes of some micro-organisms.

Together with other micro-organisms that are not commonly associated with direct aggression, such potential pathogens may share a role as opportunist invaders. It can be argued that any pathogen that exploits a weakness in a vulnerable host is opportunistic, but the term *opportunist* is currently applied to a relatively non-aggressive organism when it takes advantage of a weakened or debilitated patient. For example, man's normal defence mechanisms may be upset in drug addicts and in patients who are treated with cytotoxic drugs. It is well recognized that patients in these categories may succumb to infections with organisms that are not generally able to cause disease without the assistance of a debilitating factor to promote their attack (see p.42).

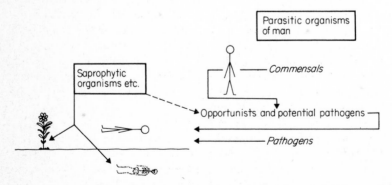

**Figure 1.2** A simplified outline: the interrelationship of saprophytes, parasites, commensals, opportunist invaders, potential pathogens and pathogens.

## SPECIES-SPECIFICITY in HOST-PARASITE ASSOCIATIONS

The pathogens that attack plants are different from those that attack animals. In turn, those that attack certain animals demonstrate affinities for specific hosts that may or may not include man. Many pathogens of man are strictly host-specific and do not naturally infect other animals. Classical examples are the typhoid bacillus, the organisms of bacillary dysentery, the diphtheria bacillus, the cholera vibrio, and the viruses of smallpox and measles. However, some organisms are pathogenic for both man and certain animals, and these are discussed in Chapter 11.

## DISEASE SYNDROMES

Patterns of signs and symptoms that characterize diseases are referred to as *syndromes*. A disease syndrome may be clearly specific for a certain disease; for example, the clinical signs and symptoms of fully developed cases of leprosy, mumps or tetanus are not likely to be confused. These particular disease syndromes are only produced as a result of infection with the leprosy bacillus, the mumps virus or the tetanus bacillus respectively, and the 'differential diagnosis' in typical cases is limited and relatively straightforward. However, the clinical syndrome associated with a simple wound infection can be produced by any one of a variety of organisms acting alone or in combination. Similarly, the clinical picture of meningitis—an infection of the central nervous system in which an ill patient has headache with neck stiffness and dislikes light shining on his eyes (photophobia)—can be produced by a meningeal infection caused by any one of several bacteria or viruses (p.55).

Thus, disease patterns are recognized in which experience teaches us to associate the probability of infection with certain ranges of organisms some of which are more likely to be involved than others. In relatively few situations, such as in leprosy or mumps or tetanus, the probabilities are essentially restricted, but the more common situation is that one of a variety of recognized causative organisms may be involved in producing an infective illness. For example, in the case of an infection of the urinary tract, the commonest pathogen is *Escherichia coli*, but urinary tract infections with *Klebsiella* species, *Streptococcus faecalis*, *Proteus* and *Pseudomonas* species, alone or in combination, are everyday occurrences (p.53). Moreover, a urinary tract infection caused by the tubercle bacillus must not be missed, and fungal and viral infections are sometimes associated with urinary tract symptoms. These special problems are dealt with elsewhere in this book. The important point is that the clinical microbiologist must restrict his search within limits demanded by practicability and experience when he attempts to isolate a causative organism and hold it responsible for a particular illness. He is often obliged to produce a reasonably accurate report as quickly as possible. It follows that he must have a considerable knowledge of the likely pathogens in a given situation. To some extent, the medical microbiologists have accordingly developed their own practical classification of bacteria and other

**Table 1.2**  A simple classification of common bacteria of medical interest.

FILAMENTOUS BACTERIA (Higher bacteria)
  *Streptomyces species* — produce various antibiotics
  *Actinomyces israelii* — causes actinomycosis

TRUE BACTERIA

| Morphology and Gram Reaction | Nature | Genus | Important infections caused by individual species | Group reference |
|---|---|---|---|---|
| Gram-positive bacilli | Aerobic | *Mycobacterium* | Tuberculosis; leprosy | Acid-fast bacilli |
| | | *Corynebacterium* | Diphtheria | Corynebacteria |
| | | *Bacillus* | Anthrax | Aerobic sporeformers |
| | Anaerobic | *Clostridium* | Tetanus; gas gangrene | Anaerobic sporeformers |
| | | *Lactobacillus** | ? | Aciduric bacilli |
| Gram-positive cocci | Aerobic | *Streptococcus* | Tonsillitis; various infections | Pyogenic cocci |
| | | *Staphylococcus* | Boils; various infections | |
| Gram-negative cocci | Aerobic | *Neisseria* | Meningitis; gonorrhoea | |
| | Anaerobic | *Veillonella* | Various infections | |
| Gram-negative bacilli | Aerobic | *Escherichia* | Various infections including wound infections and urinary tract infections | Enterobacteria |
| | | *Klebsiella* | | |
| | | *Proteus* | | |
| | | *Salmonella* | Typhoid fever; food poisoning | |
| | | *Shigella* | Bacillary dysentery | |
| | | *Pseudomonas* | Wound infections; urinary tract infection | |
| | | *Vibrio* | Cholera | |
| | | *Haemophilus* | Meningitis; respiratory tract infections | Parvobacteria |
| | | *Bordetella* | Whooping cough | |
| | | *Brucella* | Undulant fever | |
| | | *Pasteurella* | Various infections | |
| | | *Yersinia* | Plague | |
| | | *Francisella* | Tularaemia | |
| | Anaerobic | *Bacteroides* | Various infections | *Bacteroides-Fusobacterium* group |
| | | *Fusobacterium* | | |

*Strictly anaerobic lactobacilli are now in the genus *Bifidobacterium*

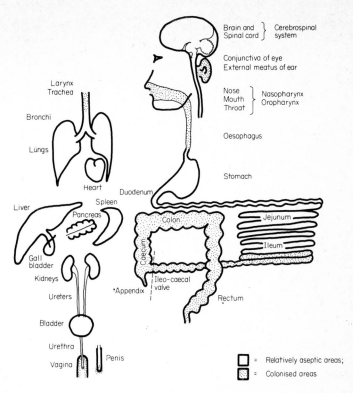

Figure 1.3   A simplified diagram of some relatively aseptic areas and colonized areas of the body. Various other aseptic areas including muscles, joints and blood vessels are omitted.

micro-organisms associated with disease in man and animals.

Simple classifications of some micro-organisms of medical importance are given on pages 1 and 4.

## COMMENSALISM

Although various antimicrobial mechanisms operate in the tissues and at epithelial surfaces to control bacterial colonization and microbial attack, there is an abundant and varied commensal flora that flourishes on the skin and on some of the mucous surfaces of the human respiratory, gastro-intestinal and genito-urinary tracts. The 'closed' systems such as the internal surfaces of joints, the cerebrospinal system, the cardiovascular system, muscles and solid organs such as the liver, spleen and brain are relatively free from bacteria and have active defence mechanisms to protect them. However, the upper respiratory tract, the terminal part of the urethra, the vagina, the mouth and throat and the terminal ileum and large bowel—and, of course, the skin—are essentially open to colonization and each has a recognized resident flora. In addition to the resident flora, other organisms may be present, usually in relatively smaller numbers, as transient flora.

**Table 1.3**    A list of aseptic and colonized areas of the body.

**Essentially sterile areas**
  Brain and spinal cord (central nervous system)
  The nervous system
  Bones, joints and muscles

**Aseptic areas** with effective clearing mechanisms
  Heart and blood vessels (cardiovascular system)
  The lymphatic system
  Lungs and terminal bronchi (lower respiratory tract)
  Liver
  Spleen
  Kidneys, ureters and bladder

**Transiently contaminated areas**
  Skin (see below)
  Conjunctiva of eye
  Upper respiratory tract (see below)
  Stomach and proximal small intestine (duodenum, jejunum, upper ileum)

**Colonized areas**
  Skin
  External meatus of ear
  Nasopharynx
         Upper respiratory tract
  Oropharynx
  Lower small bowel (terminal ileum)
  Large bowel (caecum, colon, rectum)
  Vagina
  Terminal urethra

The commensals are most numerous in the large bowel where anaerobes of the *Bacteroides-Fusobacterium* group number tens of thousands of millions ($10^{10}$) per gram of intestinal content. Here they slightly outnumber the bifidobacteria and together these groups greatly outnumber the commensal aerobic coliform organisms ($10^{6-8}$ per gram). A simplified summary of the commensal flora of man is given in Fig. 1.3 and Table 1.3.

# 2 Laboratory investigation of bacterial infection

When a bacterium produces an infective disease, it multiplies in the host and can often be isolated from the patient by various microbiological procedures that involve the culture of material submitted to the laboratory. The material may be a specimen of a discharge such as sputum, urine or faeces, or it may be frank pus. If pus is present in considerable amount, it is sent in a small sterile bottle; a swab is generally used when smaller quantities are involved. In some cases, a fragment of infected tissue removed by a surgeon may be submitted for investigation. Attention to detail in the prompt and proper submission of all such material to the laboratory is of great importance; some organisms are very susceptible to deleterious influences such as desiccation or overgrowth by more hardy commensals or contaminants; many specimens are wasted by carelessness. Special *transport media* may be used to preserve delicate organisms in transit. In some cases, special procedures are required to obtain certain samples for microbiological investigation. If it is suspected that the organism is present in the blood, samples of blood are obtained from the patient under strictly aseptic conditions and submitted in special bottles for *blood culture.* If meningitis is suspected, a sample of cerebrospinal fluid (CSF) is obtained by a procedure known as lumbar puncture and the CSF is then sent for prompt examination.

## MICROSCOPY

Some of the material submitted is usually examined promptly by microscopy, either as an unstained 'wet' preparation or, more commonly, as a stained smear. Special microscopy is sometimes required. This examination may provide direct evidence of the nature of the infecting agent; bacteria may be seen, or structures in host cells may suggest a viral infection. In addition, microscopy may provide evidence of a host reaction; for example, the presence of pus cells confirms that there is an inflammatory reaction in progress (p.28).

Despite the successful development of many special culture media and procedures, it is still not possible to grow some recognized pathogens as a routine. In other cases, the urgency of the situation demands a prompt microbiological opinion. Under these circumstances, presumptive identification may rest upon microscopic observations with the light microscope or the electronmicroscope. For example, the causative organism of syphilis may be recognized in material viewed by dark-ground microscopy, and the causative organisms of Vincent's infection of the gums or those of leprosy are not routinely cultured but may be identified on the evidence of a stained smear or tissue section. The prompt diagnosis of smallpox may be facilitated by direct electronmicroscopy.

## CULTURE PROCEDURES

Different organisms with different growth requirements are cultured on different ranges of media under various conditions. Most of the bacterial pathogens of man are grown at 37°C under aerobic conditions on nutritive media and they generally produce recognizable colonies within 24—48 hours. Some require to be grown anaerobically. Some bacteria require carbon dioxide for optimal growth. Some take several days to produce colonies and some, such as the tubercle bacillus, require several weeks.

It is sometimes relatively easy to isolate a pathogen from an ill patient by culture methods and to claim with confidence based on experience that the pathogen is the cause of the presenting illness. Most often, however, the exercise is complicated by several factors: (i) The specimen submitted may be inadequate or unsuitable, or it may have been subjected to adverse conditions in transit. (ii) The causative organism may have special growth requirements and its culture may be a demanding task, or it may be impossible to grow the pathogen with currently available procedures. (iii) The true pathogen may be present, for example in a faecal specimen or in sputum, in association with an abundant commensal flora. Careful *enrichment* and *selective* procedures are then necessary to increase the chances of isolating the 'causative organism'.

## THE KOCH-HENLE POSTULATES

The demonstration of an aetiological connection between a specific organism and a particular infective condition rests upon the above procedures. The clinician associates certain organisms with the pathogenic potential to produce a given syndrome. On the basis of past experience and a knowledge of the pathogenesis of various conditions, he develops a 'differential diagnosis' and he decides on the likely specimens to be submitted from the patient to the laboratory. The microbiologist in turn selects the range of tests most likely to demonstrate a suspected pathogen by direct (microscopical and cultural) or indirect (serological) procedures. These steps are taken almost intuitively after a period of routine clinical practice, but they relate to the postulates of Koch and Henle who first attempted to define criteria for the presumptive association of an organism with a specific disease. These workers held that the particular agent must be constantly associated with the given pathological condition and that it must be possible to recover the agent in pure culture from patients with the disease. Then it was necessary to reproduce the disease by administering the pure culture to a susceptible animal or a human volunteer. Certainly, the use of experimental animals for the demonstration of certain pathogens still has a place in diagnostic microbiology. For obvious reasons, the use of human volunteers is rather severely restricted and the use of experimental animals in Britain is very strictly controlled by law.

It will be clear that we cannot fulfil the Koch-Henle postulates for several well recognized diseases. Leprosy provides a particularly humiliating example as we can readily demonstrate the bacteria that appear to cause the disease but we cannot culture these organisms. Moreover, in diagnostic microbiology we are faced with the practical problems that (i) several different organisms may give rise to infections with similar syndromes, (ii) several different syndromes can be produced by the same organism attacking man in different ways, (iii) some non-infective diseases can initially present with a pattern that suggests a microbial cause, and (iv) the commensal flora of various sites of the body, and the healthy carrier state, confuse the situation and present many possible pitfalls. A routine laboratory approach to the examination of a specimen is illustrated in Fig. 2.1, but it should be noted that individual considerations influence the details of any such investigation.

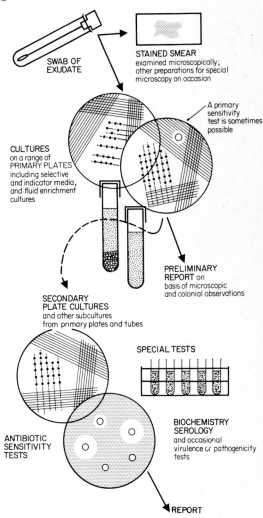

**Figure 2.1**    An outline of steps taken in bacteriological diagnosis.

In addition to procedures that attempt to meet the classical postulates, we now have the help that serological procedures can afford.

## SEROLOGY

In many but not all infective conditions, the patient develops specific *antibodies* in his serum against the infecting agent and these can be demonstrated by tests that produce observable antigen-antibody reactions in the laboratory. Examples are the agglutination test, complement-fixation tests, and various precipitin tests and neutralization tests (see below). The maximum dilution of the patient's serum at which the antibody activity is demonstrable is referred to as the *titre* of that antibody. It must be borne in mind that antibodies reacting with various organisms may be present, generally at low concentrations, in normal sera; active immunization procedures further complicate the situation. Thus, a patient may have various antibodies that are not necessarily associated with his presenting illness and some may be positively misleading. For example, a patient with a fever and a diarrhoeal illness resembling typhoid may be suffering from a form of amoebic dysentery. If the patient has been previously immunized with typhoid vaccine, a serological report will indicate that antibodies against the typhoid bacillus are present at a particular concentration. An inexperienced observer could then wrongly assume that *Salmonella typhi* is the cause of the illness. Under these circumstances, a knowledge of the previous immunization is essential and other information in the serological report can sometimes provide clues.

## SEROLOGICAL TESTS

The development of specific antimicrobial antibody in a person is indirect evidence that at some time previously the person has encountered that organism. There may be a clear history of the typical disease, but sometimes this is not so and we say that the person may have had a 'sub-clinical' or inapparent infection. Alternatively, as noted above, there may be a record of a specific artificial immunization procedure to account for the serological evidence, or, in the case of a very young child, the antibody may be passively acquired from the mother.

In the early stages of an infective illness, the demonstration of a low or insignificant level of antibody may be of positive diagnostic help. The subsequent demonstration of a *rising titre* is then good evidence that the specific organism may be involved in the current illness (Fig. 2.2). This is not always absolutely reliable, because non-specific responses sometimes occur, but it is often meaningful evidence. In a retrospective analysis of an illness, the demonstration of a *falling titre* is sometimes useful.

There are several ways in which serum antibody can be demonstrated in the laboratory for general diagnostic purposes:

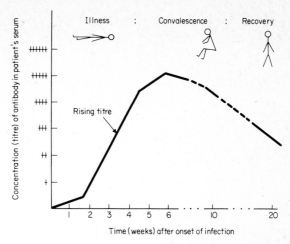

Figure 2.2    The rise and fall in antibody titre that may be demonstrable in a patient's serum.

## (1) Agglutination Tests

### (a) *Agglutination tests in tubes*

Measured aliquots of a standard suspension of the test organism are mixed with serial dilutions of the patient's serum and incubated. Agglutination can be seen as clumping of the suspension at the end of the incubation period (Fig. 2.3). The titre is the greatest dilution of the serum at which agglutination occurred. This is the principle of the Widal test for antibodies to *Salmonella typhi* (or related organisms) in the serological diagnosis of enteric fever.

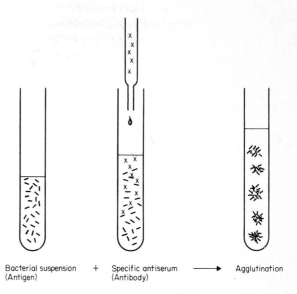

Figure 2.3    A tube agglutination test. This may also be performed as a simple slide test.

11

### (a) *Agglutination tests on slides*

Agglutinating antibodies may be demonstrated by mixing a suitable suspension of the test organism on a slide with a drop of the specific serum and rocking the mixture gently. If antibodies are present in very considerable amount, visible clumping of the organisms occurs. This procedure is used for the provisional identification of some unknown bacteria cultured from specimens and then tested against known potent specific antisera in the diagnostic laboratory, but it cannot generally be used as a direct test with patient's serum against known organisms. The principle is employed in the direct cross-matching of blood.

### (2) Precipitin Tests

When a specific antibody reacts with non-particulate soluble antigen under certain circumstances, the antigen-antibody complexes precipitate or flocculate (Fig. 2.4) and become visible as pale aggregates.

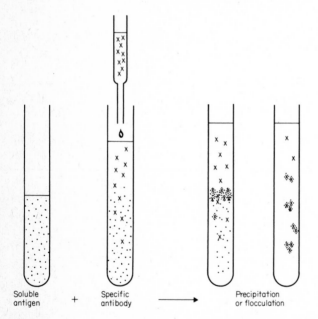

Soluble antigen    +    Specific antibody     ⟶     Precipitation or flocculation

**Figure 2.4**  A precipitin test. This principle is applied in various other procedures that may avoid the use of tubes.

### (3) Complement-fixation Tests

The complement system in serum (p.28) is involved in various antigen-antibody reactions and it is an important factor in certain associated cytolytic events. When antigen and antibody combine under certain circumstances, complement is used up or 'fixed' in the process. If a small amount of complement is available for such a reaction, it may be completely used up so that none remains for any subsequent reaction (Fig. 2.5 and q.v.).

12

*Step 1*

Patient's serum may contain (i) specific antibody (Ab) to the infecting organism, and (ii) natural complement C (in unstandarized amount).

The serum is gently heated to destroy the thermolabile natural complement.
A measured amount of guinea-pig complement C is added.

Now the patient's serum with (Ab) antibodies plus added C is mixed with specific antigen (Ag).

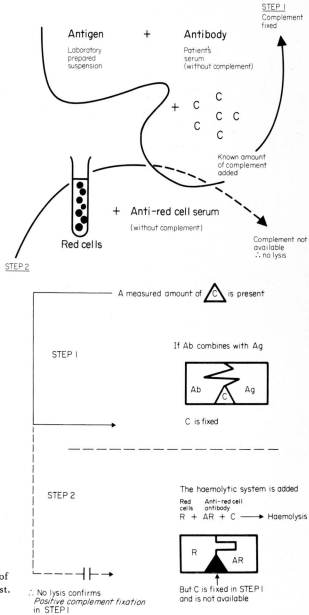

**Figure 2.5**    The principle of the complement-fixation test.

If an antigen and antibody are present together in the presence of comp-lement, the latter will be consumed. If either the antigen or the antibody is absent, complement will not be consumed. The whole purpose then is to establish whether complement has, or has not, been consumed, and that is the second stage of the test:

*Step 2*

Test for C by adding another antigen-antibody system (a 'haemolytic system') comprising sheep red cells (R) and anti-sheep red cell serum (AR) that has been heated (to render it free from natural C).

This mixture needs C to cause lysis of the sheep red cells. If the reaction in Step 1 was positive however, C is not available for Step 2. The red cells remain unlysed. In terms of Step 1, the diagnostic test, this represents a *positive result.*

### (4)  Neutralization tests and related tests

Certain antigens produce demonstrable effects in animals or in-vitro systems. For instance, some toxic bacterial proteins ('toxins') may be lethal or haemolytic, and some viruses may attack cells in culture (cytopathic effect) or may cause red cells to stick together (haemagglutination). Specific anti-bodies prepared against these various agents may inhibit or neutralize these demonstrable reactions and this is the basis of specific serological neutralization or inhibition tests (Fig. 2.6).

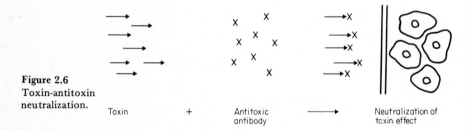

**Figure 2.6**
Toxin-antitoxin
neutralization.

Toxin          +          Antitoxic          ⟶          Neutralization of
                                  antibody                          toxin effect

### (5)  Immunofluorescence procedures

Certain dyes such as fluorescein that fluoresce when exposed to ultraviolet light are used in various ways to label antibody:
(i)     In some cases, *direct* labelling is of diagnostic use.
For example, a specific antiserum prepared against a surface somatic antigen of a bacterial cell may be conjugated with fluorescein. A dried smear of exudate or culture thought to contain the bacterium is then treated with the conjugated antiserum and, if the specific bacterium is present, the labelled antiserum sticks to it and is not lost during a final washing stage. The bacterium is then seen to fluoresce when the smear is viewed by ultraviolet light in a specially equipped microscope.
(ii)    In other cases, *indirect* labelling is used.

14

Here, the initially applied antibody is not labelled but the smear containing the antigen goes through a further procedure after being exposed to the specific antibody. A special (labelled) antiserum prepared against the globulin of the species used for the preparation of the specific antiserum is applied and this fixes the fluorescent label to the specific antibody that has located its antigen in the smear. There are various permutations of this principle.

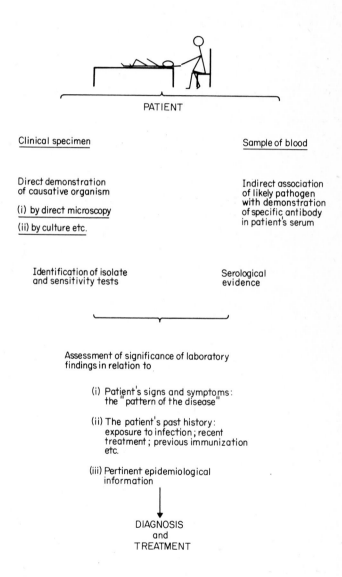

**Figure 2.7**   Medical microbiology in relation to the diagnosis and treatment of infection.

15

# 3 Pathogenic viruses

These non-cellular obligately intracellular parasites are mentioned in Volume 1 of this series (page 26) and described in detail in Volume 2. The basic chemical components of the virus particle or *virion* are protein and either DNA or RNA, but both forms of nucleic acid do not occur in any one virus. The DNA is usually double-stranded and the RNA is usually single-stranded, though exceptions occur in each of these cases.

Whether viruses should be considered as parasitic entities or bits of rogue nucleic acid is debatable. The capacity of many viruses to be transmitted to a new host and there to upset the metabolism of various human cells and to redirect the host cell metabolic pathways to the reproduction of virions makes this aspect of microbiology of great significance in the study of infectious disease. The capacity of some viruses to change host cell metabolism in more subtle and less directly expressed ways is of interest in many related medical fields including the study of familial diseases, medical genetics and cancer.

## THE LABORATORY DIAGNOSIS OF VIRAL INFECTIONS

### Microscopy

Under certain circumstances, a pathogenic virus may be recognized and a presumptive diagnosis made on the basis of direct electronmicroscopy of material derived from a patient. This can be done in the case of smallpox when the typical virions may be seen in preparations of material obtained from the skin vesicles. The procedure may be of considerable value in distinguishing promptly between an atypical case of chickenpox and smallpox.

In other circumstances, light microscopy of stained host cells may reveal appearances associated with specific viral infection. For example, the virus of rabies produces typical eosinophilic inclusion bodies (Negri bodies) in the cytoplasm of nerve cells in the brain; this finding made at autopsy on a dog can be of immediate medical value and calls for action to be taken to protect those that may have been in contact with the animal. Cells obtained from the lesions of smallpox patients similarly show eosinophilic intracytoplasmic inclusions (Guarnieri bodies). Cells affected by herpesviruses show intranuclear inclusions and there may be giant cell formation.

Immunofluorescence procedures are being increasingly developed for the specific identification of viruses in host cells and it is in this field and in the observation of cytopathic effects *in vitro* (q.v.) that the light microscope is most likely to be of prompt service in diagnostic virology.

16

## Isolation and culture procedures

A pathogenic virus may be isolated from infected material submitted to the laboratory by seeding a suitable substrate of living cells and ultimately harvesting and identifying the product. Viruses cannot replicate independently of a host cell and each virus has a clearly specific affinity for a certain range of host cells. The range is determined *inter alia* by the nature of receptor sites on the host cell surface and by the properties of the particular virus protein coat. A suitable cell culture system may be one of the following: (1) an experimental animal, or (2) a fertile egg (chick embryo), or (3) an in-vitro culture of tissue cells (cell or tissue culture), or (4) an in-vitro culture of an intact segment of differentiated tissue (organ culture).

Animals are not frequently used now for the primary detection of many viruses, whereas cell cultures are used as a routine for many isolations. Dispersed cells from fragments of certain human or animal tissues are generally cultured in monolayers adherent to the internal walls of glass test-tubes. The cells are bathed in a nutrient fluid and the tubes are usually rotated during incubation. If the cells are suitable for the growth of the virus, the events that follow addition of the infective material are as follows. First, a virus particle (virion) may adsorb to the host cell surface and then, perhaps by a process called pinocytosis, it enters the host cell. Now the virion loses its protein coat (capsid) and the uncoated viral nucleic acid is released. At this stage, the virus is essentially undetectable and this is called the *eclipse phase*. However, the viral genome (genetic material) proceeds to specify all of the components

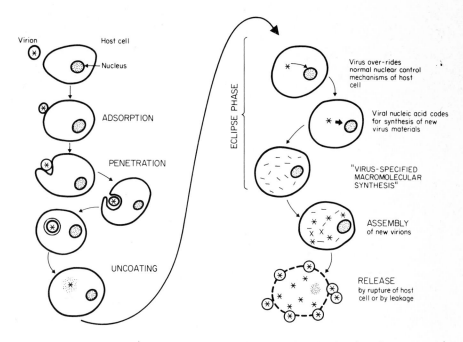

**Figure 3.1**    Stages of viral infection and replication (not drawn to scale).

17

required for new virus to be assembled, and the host cell metabolism is thus taken over and redirected to the production of virions (Fig. 3.1).

Cells supporting viral multiplication may or may not show signs that all is not well with them. There may be obvious damage and cell death—a *cytopathic effect* (CPE) (Fig. 3.2), or there may be a tendency to overgrowth (hyperplasia),

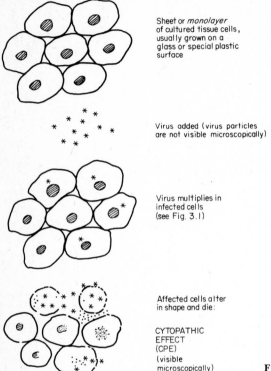

Sheet or *monolayer* of cultured tissue cells, usually grown on a glass or special plastic surface

Virus added (virus particles are not visible microscopically)

Virus multiplies in infected cells (see Fig. 3.1)

Affected cells alter in shape and die:

CYTOPATHIC EFFECT (CPE) (visible microscopically)

**Figure 3.2**  Virus cytopathic effect.

sometimes with changes of a malignant nature. Some cells infected with certain viruses and supporting their multiplication show no visible change. If a monolayer of cells is treated with a virus preparation diluted so that only a proportion of the cells are infected and if the monolayer is overlaid with a semi-solid medium, any visible cytopathic effect is then localized to the area of the initially infected cell; the released virus successively attacks contiguous cells and is not randomly disseminated as it would be in a fluid culture system. The result is that *plaques* (punched-out areas) of degenerate cells develop in the monolayer and these areas show up clearly when the monolayer is stained with a dye.

**Characterization and identification**

The identification of a particular virus depends upon obtaining evidence in

18

Table 3.1 Some viruses of medical interest.

| | Type of nucleic acid | Group name | Examples | Disease Produced |
|---|---|---|---|---|
| Ortho-myxoviruses | RNA | The Myxoviruses | Influenza A, B and C viruses | Influenza |
| Para-myxoviruses | RNA | | Mumps virus<br>Measles virus | Mumps<br>Measles |
| Picornaviruses | RNA | The Enteroviruses | Polioviruses (types 1—3)<br>Coxsackie viruses<br>Echoviruses | Poliomyelitis<br>Meningitis, pleurodynia, myocarditis<br>Meningitis, diarrhoea |
| | | | Rhinoviruses | Coryza |
| Rhabdoviruses | RNA | | Rabies virus | Rabies |
| Togaviruses | RNA | The Arboviruses* | Group A<br>Group B<br><br>Group C | Encephalitis<br>Yellow fever, dengue fever, louping ill, encephalitis.<br>Encephalitis |
| Adenoviruses | DNA | | Adenovirus (types 1—31) | Respiratory tract infections |
| Herpesviruses | DNA | | Herpesvirus hominis<br><br>Varicella-zoster virus | Herpes simplex (stomatitis, 'cold sores', etc.)<br>Chickenpox, Herpes zoster (shingles) |
| Papovaviruses | DNA | | Papilloma viruses | Warts |
| Poxviruses | DNA | | Variola virus<br>Vaccinia virus used as vaccine against smallpox; is related to virus of cowpox. | Smallpox |

* Other arboviruses belong to different virus groups (see p.83).

19

some of the following categories:

(i)   *Morphology*: Electronmicroscopy of suitably stained preparations may reveal details of shape or structure that are helpful in classification.

(ii)   *Range of susceptible cells*: Viruses vary in their affinities for different host cells and this information may provide a useful clue.

(iii)   *Appearances in culture systems*: The reaction of the fertile egg to a virus, as in the production of pocks in response to an inoculation of a poxvirus, may be of diagnostic value. The reaction of an in-vitro cell culture system may also provide evidence of diagnostic value revealed by light microscopy of stained preparations. In some cases, the cytopathic effect may itself have appearances that provide clues.

(iv)   *Special reactions*: For example, *haemagglutination* and *haemadsorption*. Some viruses, notably the orthomyxoviruses and paramyxoviruses have affinity for certain mucoproteins (glycoproteins) at cell surfaces. This can be demonstrated by their ability to adhere to the surface of red blood cells and to cause them to agglutinate (haemagglutination).

(v)   *Effects produced in the experimental animal*: In some cases, reproduction of a disease syndrome or the production of a particular histopathological effect in the tissues of an experimental animal may indicate the identity of the virus.

(vi)   *Serology*: The identification of an isolated virus is often clinched by serological evidence. A suspension of the cultured virus may be shown to react specifically with an antiserum prepared against a known virus. This may depend upon a *precipitin reaction* (see p.12) or a *complement-fixation* reaction (see pp.12–14). In some cases it is possible to show that a specific antiserum will protect a cell culture system against a cytopathic effect or an animal against a pathogenic effect; these are referred to as *neutralization tests*.

If the virus has haemagglutinating properties, specific serological *haemagglutination-inhibition* can be demonstrated, provided that non-specific inhibitors are first removed from the serum by chemical or enzymic methods.

It should be noted that viruses abound in nature and they may be encountered by chance in tissue or secretions submitted from a patient with a disease quite unrelated to that particular virus. Just as the bacteriologist must be on guard to distinguish a commensal organism from an active pathogen, the virologist must be aware of the existence of latent or passenger viruses in tissues. Moreover, the virologist has the additional problem of dealing with cell culture systems which are themselves contaminated from time to time with bacteria or fungi or viruses or mycoplasmas. Bacterial and fungal contamination can be recognized without undue difficulty, but the other potential contaminants can occasionally produce a bewildering series of false clues in diagnostic and experimental virology.

# 4 Medical mycology

As far as we know, most of the vast numbers of different fungi that occur in nature cause no harm to man. Some are of great use and we have exploited them in baking and in brewing, in cheese-making, in the chemical industry, in various manufacturing processes, and in the production of some of our most valuable antimicrobial agents.

A few fungi are recognized as pathogens of man and animals. In general, fungal elements in the tissues do not seem to excite the dramatic sort of host reactions that are typically associated with some bacterial or viral infections, though people sensitized to various fungi may sometimes respond acutely to a fungal infection or to inhalation of fungal elements in the air. The avenues of mycological infection are relatively restricted to the respiratory route and to skin contact often with the assistance of minor injury.

The pathogenic fungi include those that cause systemic infections or 'deep mycoses' and those typically associated with epidermal infections—'superficial mycoses'—affecting tissues such as skin, hair or nail.

## DEEP MYCOSES

### 1. Meningeal involvement
The ovoid yeast-like fungus *Cryptococcus neoformans* occurs in bird droppings. It may be inhaled and causes various forms of disease in man including a meningeal infection involving the brain.

### 2. Respiratory involvement
*Blastomyces dermatitidis* is also acquired by the respiratory route. It is a *dimorphic* fungus, i.e. it occurs as a yeast-like form in the tissues or under certain conditions *in vitro*, but it can also occur in a mycelial form. Blastomycosis may affect various tissues and organs; it typically involves the lungs.

*Coccidioides immitis* is a dimorphic fungus that usually affects the lungs after its airborne spores have been inhaled.

*Histoplasma capsulatum*, another dimorphic fungus occurring in soil and dust, can cause respiratory disease that may resemble tuberculosis.

### 3. Deep cutaneous involvement
Various fungi are associated with deep skin infections that may be very disfiguring and disabling. Sporotrichosis is caused by *Sporotrichum schenckii* and is characterized by the formation of a pustule at the site of a minor injury with extension to regional lymph nodes and abscess formation. Chromoblastomycosis is a similar syndrome caused by other fungi. Mycetoma or Madura foot are

terms used to describe nodular necrotic lesions with suppuration and sinus formation caused by a variety of filamentous fungi and seen quite frequently in tropical countries.

## SUPERFICIAL MYCOSES

### 1. Superficial involvement of mucosal surfaces

The yeast-like fungus *Candida albicans* (*Monilia albicans*) is a commensal of the mouth; it produces a superficial infection commonly of the mucosa of the vagina or the mouth where its speckled white appearance on the dark epithelial surface has given rise to the term 'thrush' for this condition. Thrush frequently occurs in the mouths of young children, and vaginal thrush is very common in women of childbearing age and in later years. As the condition is often associated with a local or general lowering of tissue resistance, *C. albicans* has been described as a better index of the early development of abnormality than the chemical tests on which clinicians rely. This is an overstatement, but it underlines the typical association of *Candida* infection with some predisposing factor such as immaturity, pregnancy, diabetes, nutritional deficiency, steroid therapy, leukaemia and other malignant states, or local tissue damage. The fungus can infect the nail fold of a finger and give rise to a condition called paronychia and it can also affect nail tissue. *Candida* may be quick to take advantage of the suppression of the local commensal flora by broad-spectrum antibiotic therapy and a generalized spread may then involve the gastro-intestinal tract or the respiratory system.

### 2. Superficial involvement of skin, nails and hair: The dermatophytes

Filamentous fungi of the genera *Microsporum*, *Trichophyton* and *Epidermophyton* cause infections affecting skin, nails and hair. The causative organisms attack keratin and the associated infections characteristically remain superficial. The centrifugal spreading appearance of the advancing edge of the lesion in the skin earned it the term *ringworm*; a synonym is *tinea*. The fungi involved are collectively called the dermatophytes.

Some of the ringworm fungi are anthropophilic, being primarily associated with man, whereas zoophilic species primarily infect animals and are occasionally transmitted to man. The primary habitat of geophilic species is the soil; some pathogenic ringworm fungi of man can certainly persist for many weeks in soil, but it is doubtful whether soil is a true primary source for these organisms.

*Microsporum audouinii* and *M. canis* cause scalp ringworm, *tinea capitis*, in school children; the affected hairs are broken off and a circular patch of erythematous scaling or encrusted scalp is seen. The condition is contagious and may be transmitted via combs and brushes. If a zoophilic *Trichophyton* species is acquired from a calf or a pony, the affected area may show a more vigorous response with pus formation and painful swelling.

Ringworm of the body, *tinea corporis*, often affects the groin or the skin

22

between the toes (athlete's foot), and the causative fungus may be *Epidermophyton floccosum*.

*M. canis*, *T. rubrum*, *T. mentagrophytes* and *T. verrucosum* are species that may also cause body ringworm, and some of these may affect nail tissue.

## MISCELLANEOUS FUNGAL CONDITIONS

Some fungi involved occasionally in human disease are on the borderline between the saprophytic and the pathogenic state. For example, *Aspergillus fumigatus* may gain access to an area of diseased or devitalized lung tissue in a person affected by some other disease. The fungus may grow virtually saprophytically in the affected tissues under these circumstances to produce an 'aspergilloma' that may require specific therapy to control its further development.

Some saprophytic actinomycetes and fungi may produce heavy concentrations of spores or mycelial fragments that can become airborne under certain conditions and may be inhaled in significant amounts. Repeated exposure to these fungal antigens can result in the development of antibodies that may precipitate various local hypersensitivity reactions affecting the respiratory tract. This type of illness is now recognized as an occupational hazard for workers in various industries and the syndromes are accordingly known by such terms as farmer's lung, maple bark stripper's disease and maltworker's disease.

## FUNGAL TOXINS (MYCOTOXINS)

Toxic substances produced by *Aspergillus flavus* and called aflatoxins are of considerable biological interest. These toxins interfere with DNA synthesis and they have mutagenic and carcinogenic potential. For example, aflatoxins administered to animals have been shown to cause a form of liver cancer (hepatoma). They may be produced in mouldy materials destined for animal or poultry feeding and this has caused trouble; on a much smaller scale they have been incriminated in human disease in underdeveloped areas. Various other toxic fungal products are known and some of these are associated with toxic syndromes in animals.

## LABORATORY DIAGNOSIS OF FUNGAL DISEASE

The diagnosis of deep fungal infections depends upon microscopical examination and culture of secretions and affected tissue submitted from the patient, together with serological evidence that may be available in some cases.

The mycological diagnosis of ringworm infections rests upon the microscopical evidence of smears or sections of infected tissues and the microscopical and naked-eye appearance of cultures derived from that material. Serological tests are not used.

*Candida* infections are readily diagnosed by examination of stained smears (Fig. 4.1) and by culture of the causative organism from swabs or affected tissue. The species is determined by various cultural tests. *C. albicans* is the commonest, but other species are sometimes involved.

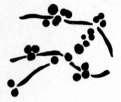

**Figure 4.1**   *Candida albicans*—a yeast-like fungus that causes superficial infections of mucous membranes.

## THE LABORATORY CULTURE OF FUNGI

Fungi and yeasts are generally cultured at temperatures in the 20–28°C range. They grow more slowly than bacteria and usually require some days or weeks to produce fully developed colonies. Mycological cultures are always grown aerobically and usually on carbohydrate-rich media with antibacterial agents added to exclude bacterial contamination.

The ringworm fungi can be conveniently cultured on a small segment of a suitable agar medium sandwiched between a microscope slide and a coverslip (Fig. 4.2). The edge of the medium is seeded with the fungus and the preparation is incubated in a petri dish with damp filter paper to prevent desiccation

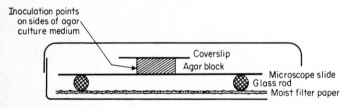

**Figure 4.2**   A needle mount preparation suitable for the culture of fungi for subsequent microscopic examination.

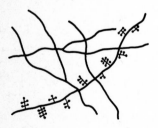

**Figure 4.3**   Diagrammatic representation of fungal hyphae showing **micro**conidia. (X *c.* 400).

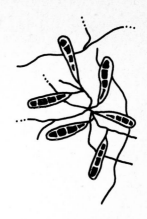

**Figure 4.4**  Diagrammatic representation of fungal hyphae showing **macro**conidia. (X *c.* 500).

of the agar block. In due course, fungal hyphae grow and extend on to the adjacent glass surfaces. They interlace to produce a mycelium and develop various special structures such as *microconidia* or *macroconidia* typical of different species (Figs. 4.3 and 4.4). These structures are well demonstrated by removing the agar block and staining the material that is adherent to the slide and coverslip with lactophenol blue; two preparations can be made by matching a clean slide with the fungus-covered coverslip and a clean coverslip with the original slide. The microscopic appearances revealed in this way, the colonial appearances of cultures grown on agar surfaces in plates or flat bottles, and the reactions of pure cultures in biochemical tests, distinguish the different genera and species.

# 5 Host defence systems and the immune response

**IMMUNITY**

Man's ability to defend himself against infection by potentially pathogenic organisms depends in the first instance on the integrity of various body surfaces such as the skin and the epithelial surfaces of the eyes, and the respiratory, gastro-intestinal and genito-urinary systems. The defences of these areas are supplemented by the local production of various antimicrobial factors. For instance, the skin has antibacterial fatty acids and the gastric acid of the stomach acts as an effective antimicrobial barrier. The action of the eyelids and the production of tears containing lysozyme produces an antimicrobial flushing action, and the presence of mucus together with peristaltic activity in the gut—or ciliary activity at some points in the respiratory tract—combine to repel and expel potential invaders. In some areas, the local commensal microbial flora (p.5) plays an important part in the defensive complex. The special flora of the adult vagina, for example, is associated with the maintenance of a locally protective acid reaction.

Our resistance to infection is further dependent upon systems that operate in our blood and tissue-fluids to cope with organisms that may, from time to time, get past the first line of defence. Antimicrobial factors in the blood include basic proteins that inactivate some organisms and specific antibodies that develop in response to infection. A most important defensive system at this level involves the white blood cells. Polymorphonuclear leucocytes or *'polymorphs'*, so-called because their nuclei are lobulate, have the power to engulf or ingest foreign particles; i.e., they are phagocytic and, having taken a bacterial cell in they may bring to bear on it various hydrolytic enzymes to kill and digest it. A chemotactic system operates by which these phagocytic cells are attracted by chemical mediators liberated at the site of infection and this allows them to home on to the target. Polymorphs can deal to some extent with bacteria in this manner at the host's first encounter with a new invader, but they can deal much more effectively if the organisms become coated with specific antibody. This is referred to as an opsonic effect. Some pathogens may resist digestion within the phagocyte and, in turn, may kill the polymorph. Dead polymorphs, degraded tissue and fibrinous material are referred to as pus, and bacteria that provoke such a reaction are referred to as pyogenic (p.28).

Other phagocytic cells with simple large nuclei occur in the blood where they are called monocytes; they can leave the circulation and act as *wandering macrophages* (large phagocytes) in the tissues. Similar cells present in the walls of blood vessels in various tissues are referred to as *fixed macrophages*. The job

26

of the macrophages is essentially to pick up and digest foreign particulate matter—at which they are remarkably efficient—and in some cases they present antigenic material to *lymphocytes*. The lymphocytes are white blood cells involved in the initiation of the immune response which takes two forms. In one form, certain lymphocytes differentiate to *plasma cells* that produce specific antibody. This is the basis of our *humoral immunity*. The transformation of a lymphocyte into a plasma cell is triggered by antigen and other factors. When pathogenic bacteria gain access to the host's tissues in significant numbers, the organisms act as complex antigens and stimulate the production of various antibodies (immunoglobulins) by these transformed lymphocytes. The antibodies may then react with the organisms in various ways (p.10), generally to the disadvantage of the invader. These antibodies present in the blood serum (humoral antibodies) may react against some component of the body of a bacterium (somatic anti-O antibodies) or against appendages such as flagella (flagellar anti-H antibodies) and they may be specifically antibacterial or antiviral or antitoxic. Other lymphocytes are involved in a less clearly defined but important and related system that operates at the cellular level by direct action on infected, altered or damaged host cells. This is called *cell-mediated immunity*.

Lymphocytes involved in the above systems have a common origin in primitive stem cells in the foetal liver and in the spleen and bone marrow. Two classes are recognized: The *B lymphocytes* are derived from cells in the bone marrow and are influenced by intestinal lymphoid tissue; the B cells are primarily concerned with the production of IgM and later IgG antibody (see below) when they are transformed by antigen. The *T lymphocytes* are essentially matured in and influenced by the thymus. They co-operate with B lymphocytes in various ways, but T lymphocytes are particularly associated with the cell-mediated immune system.

### The Immunoglobulins

These substances, referred to on p.107, are involved in specific immune reactions. They are a group of serum proteins and five classes can be distinguished (see Fig. 5.1):

*Immunoglobulin M* (IgM) is produced early in the host response to antigen and is involved in agglutination, opsonization, complement-fixation and lytic reactions.

*Immunoglobulin G* (IgG), the major component, is produced relatively late in the host's response to a new antigen. It is involved in precipitation reactions, antitoxin (neutralization) activity, and complement-fixation reactions.

*Immunoglobulin A* (IgA) occurs in serum, but it is also typically associated with local antibody production at mucous surfaces where, in conjunction with a 'secretory piece' which allows its secretion across the mucous membrane, it appears to play a protective role. It is present in the respiratory tract, the gut, and the urinary tract, and it occurs in human milk, tears and saliva.

*Immunoglobulin E* (IgE) has affinity for host cell surfaces and seems to be involved in hypersensitivity reactions and allergy.

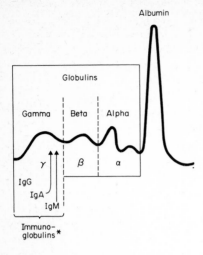

**Figure 5.1**    Protein components of serum distinguishable by electrophoresis.

*Immunoglobulin D* (IgD) does not have a clearly recognized role.

### Complement

This is a complex system of serum proteins involved in various antigen-antibody reactions. When it is activated by such a reaction *in vivo*, it has lytic activity for cell membranes and this may be brought to bear on Gram-negative bacteria—rendering them vulnerable to lysozyme—or on host tissue cells. The complement system is also involved in chemotaxis and in hypersensitivity reactions. It is also thought to be responsible for ·some of the features of bacteriogenic shock (p.41).

### ACUTE INFLAMMATION—The pyogenic response

Various forms of tissue injury elicit an acute inflammatory response. This is a commonly observed tissue reaction to a chemical injury, or to a burn, or to a local infection in the skin, and it may also occur in other tissues when an infection localizes, for example in the lung. The blood vessels are primarily involved and the reactions are classically described in relation to events that can be seen in the skin. After a very transient vasoconstrictive effect there is a sustained local increase in blood supply, resulting from dilatation of the capillary vessels in the area; this causes a visible flush or erythema. The vascular changes are mediated initially by local histamine release and thereafter by other chemicals liberated at the site. In turn, fluid in the capillaries escapes through widened spaces between the cells lining the blood vessels and accumulates in greater amounts than is usual. A tetrad of rubor, calor, tumor and dolor

28

(redness, warmth, swelling and pain) results. The fluid is subsequently reabsorbed by the capillary network and by lymphatic pathways that channel it back to the venous system, but this takes time. Meanwhile, polymorph leucocytes are first attracted from the blood circulating through the local vessels. They move out of the mainstream to the altered cell surface lining the affected vessels (margination) and then pass between those cells into the tissue where chemotaxis operates. At a later stage, mononuclear cells (macrophages) emigrate from the blood in response to these changes and take over the main phagocytic function leading to clearance and repair (resolution).

## PUS: PYOGENS AND PYROGENS

A mixture of dead polymorphs, necrotic tissue and degraded blood products constitutes pus. If this is localized in a tissue, it is an abscess. Sometimes small abscesses can be resolved by natural processes of scavenging by macrophages and repair by tissue regeneration or by the laying down of fibrous tissue (scar formation). In relatively superficial sites, abscesses may 'point' and discharge as a boil does, but it is sometimes necessary to expedite this by surgical intervention to remove the frank pus. This relieves pressure in the tissues and thus reduces pain and accelerates healing. Moreover, the absorption of various toxic products from a local abscess may give rise to various 'constitutional upsets' that include fever, malaise and headache. Many of us appreciate the general and local misery of a dental abscess and can testify to the relief obtained by an admittedly worrying operation to secure drainage. Fever associated with an infection is a general effect attributed to the absorption of a *pyrogenic* agent, not to be confused with the local *pyogenic* effect that is described above. The pyrogen is thought to be a host factor released from damaged phagocytes and is sometimes referred to as endogenous pyrogen; this operates via the brain and a prostaglandin mediator.

## CHRONIC INFLAMMATORY REACTIONS

The body's reactions to some pathogens are not typically acute. This partly relates to the type of pathogen, partly to the state of immunity of the host, and partly to other factors in the host.

For example, although an early response to a first encounter with the tubercle bacillus in the tissues of a child or young adult may have the features of a mild acute inflammation, the subsequent reaction does not develop as a classical acute response to pyogenic organisms. Monocyte-derived macrophages surround the infected zone and there is a central area of dead (necrotic) material that does not liquefy into frank pus, but is usually referred to as a zone of caseation or of cheese-like material. The macrophages assume two forms: flattened 'epithelioid cells' (quite unrelated to epithelial cells) and large multinucleate 'giant cells'. These are joined at the periphery of the lesion during the ensuing weeks by fibroblasts and lymphocytes. In time, the cellularity of the peripheral zone declines, the viable bacterial content progressively diminishes, and a sterile calcified structure may ultimately mark the site of the battle. In many cases, however, viable tubercle bacilli may remain for many years and there may be a recrudescence of disease with spread from this site.

## INTRALEUCOCYTIC KILLING

When a leucocyte has ingested an organism, the cell is then programmed for inactivation and digestion of the engulfed microbe. The basic steps are illustrated in Fig. 5.2. Oxygen consumption increases and lactic acid accumulates; the hexose-monophosphate shunt is boosted, and there is an increase in the production of hydrogen peroxide. The lysosomes are activated during the stage of *degranulation*; the intracytoplasmic granular appearance of the leucocyte diminishes as the lysosomes fuse with the phagosome where their digestive hydrolases and antibacterial cationic proteins are brought to bear on the ingested particle.

CHEMOTAXIS

ENGULFMENT (PHAGOCYTOSIS)

PARTICLE NOW WITHIN PHAGOSOME

DEGRANULATION; FUSION OF LYSOSOMES WITH PHAGOSOME

DIGESTION OF PARTICLE

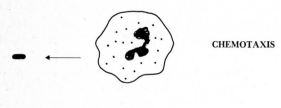

**Figure 5.2**    Chemotaxis, engulfment, phagocytosis and intraleucocytic digestion.

30

Leucocytes are rich in myeloperoxidase which is actively microbicidal in the presence of locally produced peroxide and a halogen co-factor. Iron-binding proteins present in serum and in some leucocyte fractions are bacteriostatic when not fully saturated with iron; and lysozyme, in conjunction with the complement system activated by specific antibody, attacks bacterial cell walls and renders cell membranes vulnerable.

## HOST DEFICIENCIES OR DEFECTS

A patient may be at a serious quantitative or qualitative disadvantage in his capacity to cope with an infecting organism.

Patients receiving treatment with certain drugs or radiations—including such substances as cytotoxic agents for the control of neoplastic disease, chloramphenicol for a severe infection, phenylbutazone for a rheumatoid condition, or X-ray therapy—may have infective complications that result from suppression of the production or activity of their leucocytes.

Some children are born with an inherited inability to produce immunoglobulins (agammaglobulinaemia) or with a significantly restricted ability to do so (hypogammaglobulinaemia). Their cell-mediated immune mechanisms work, but they are unduly vulnerable to infections with pyogenic bacteria in which our humoral defence systems play important roles. Other children with an inherited disease called chronic granulomatous disease of childhood have a defect in their intraleucocytic killing system and they are unduly susceptible to attack by certain bacteria, notably staphylococci and coliform bacilli, and fungi such as *Candida*, which they cannot control.

# 6 Bacterial pathogenicity

### Components of Pathogenicity

The various components involved in the expression of bacterial pathogenicity have been summarized as follows. The *source* of the infectious agent may be a human or animal case of the disease or a carrier. There is then a stage of *transmission* of the infectious challenge to the new host, followed by a process during which the *infectivity* of the agent is expressed. Thereafter, the organism damages the host and expresses its virulence by essentially invasive or toxic mechanisms or a combination of these (see Fig. 6.1).

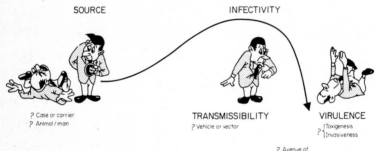

SOURCE           INFECTIVITY

? Case or carrier
? Animal / man

TRANSMISSIBILITY
? Vehicle or vector

? Avenue of infection

VIRULENCE
? {Toxigenesis, Invasiveness}

**Figure 6.1**   Factors in pathogenicity.

The outcome of such an attack on a new host depends upon many variables that may influence the host-parasite association.

### Measurement of challenge doses

In experimental work, we consider infective hazards in qualitative terms and also in relation to the size of the challenge dose that may produce some demonstrable effect.

A simple concept, at least in theory, is the minimum lethal dose (MLD) for a specified test animal. In practice, as animal and human responses to infective or toxic challenges vary so much among individuals, the MLD is not a reliable measurement. It is better to work in terms of the LD50, the dose that is lethal for 50 per cent of a test group of similar animals. If the standard indicating effect is not death but some other result, we work in terms of the effective dose (ED) and the ED50. The ID50 is similarly used if infectivity is measured. There is no need to be restricted to 50 per cent in these measurements; the ED75 or the ED35 might be of interest. However, it is well known that dose-response curves tend to be linear in their mid-section and are far from linear at the extremes where individual variation is so obvious.

In experimental work, therefore, we are seldom concerned with the ED1, the effective dose for 1 per cent of the test group; and we are even less concerned with the dose that might affect 0.01 per cent of the test group. On the other hand, those who are responsible for the production and distribution of our processed foods for example, realize that they have in Britain a potential test group of 50 million individuals. An ED1 challenge in a widely distributed food under these circumstances would be catastrophic. Moreover, it will be clear that a human population is in no way composed of similar individuals. Susceptibility to various bacterial challenges in such a group varies enormously, and there are innumerable permutations of circumstances that might influence the challenges. We must take into account various factors that influence the nature and size of an infective challenge, the avenue or route by which it is delivered, and the susceptibility or resistance of the recipient who may become the new host.

## SOURCES OF INFECTION: CASES AND CARRIER STATES: SPREAD OF INFECTION

### The Source
The ultimate source of an infection is the site in the human, animal, plant or soil in which the causative organism naturally thrives.

### The Case
The usual source of many infections of man is often another human being who may be a clinically apparent case of the disease, excreting or exhaling the organism into the environment or passing it on by close contact.

Just after the early incubation period of many diseases, the infected person may be highly infectious and this is often the stage when the victim has not yet 'gone down' with the infection, has not yet called for medical help, and has not yet advised friends to keep away.

### The Convalescent Carrier
When a patient is recovering from an infection, he may continue to shed potentially infective organisms into the environment.

In some cases, notably in typhoid fever, a *chronic carrier state* may persist indefinitely.

### The Healthy Carrier
We are all healthy carriers of potentially dangerous commensal organisms, and this is discussed below in relation to endogenous infection. For example, the *Escherichia coli* organisms of our intestinal flora can cause diarrhoeal disease if they are introduced under suitable conditions into susceptible hosts. The staphylococci that many of us carry in our noses are equally versatile and potentially dangerous to our colleagues and contacts.

### Animal Sources of Infection

Diseases transmitted to man from animals are called zoonoses. They are described in Chapter 11.

### Sources of Infection in Soil

Some fungal pathogens of man can grow in soil, and some bacterial pathogens excreted by man and animals, for example the anaerobic spore-forming clostridia of gas-gangrene and tetanus, may survive and multiply in warm manured soil under certain conditions.

## TERMINOLOGY

Inanimate objects involved in the transfer of infection are sometimes referred to as *fomites*, and indirect transfer of infection may be by so-called mediate contact (q.v.). The study of aspects of the incidence and spread of infection—dealing with the time, the place and the persons involved—is called *epidemiology*.

An infection is said to be *endemic* if it occurs relatively constantly in an area. It is said to be *epidemic* when its incidence increases sharply to involve large numbers of people in an area, and *pandemic* when it spreads in epidemic proportions across continents.

In Britain, bacillary dysentery and streptococcal sore throat are endemic diseases. There are occasional epidemics of influenza, and this disease sometimes becomes alarmingly pandemic.

### Endogenous and Exogenous Infection

When a component of the commensal flora attacks its host, the infection is said to be *endogenous*. This can happen, for example, when an abdominal wound penetrates a colonized area of the bowel or when a potentially pathogenic staphylococcus carried in the nose is allowed to gain access to a wound on the hand. There are many other circumstances in which an endogenous infection may occur.

An *exogenous* infection is said to occur when the pathogen is acquired directly from another person or animal or indirectly via some object or item of furniture.

## TRANSMISSION: AVENUES OR ROUTES OF INFECTION

Unless a particular pathogen is brought to a susceptible host by a route that allows access to a vulnerable system for that pathogen, the typical infection will not be produced and, in many cases, an infection will not be established at all (see Fig. 6.2). For example, tetanus bacilli are not infective by ingestion, and cholera organisms do not naturally infect through skin or by an airborne route.

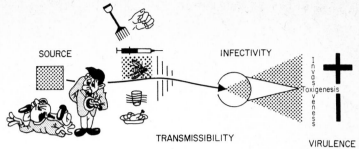

SOURCE INFECTIVITY

Invasiveness

Toxigenesis

TRANSMISSIBILITY

VIRULENCE

**Figure 6.2**    Components of pathogenicity.

### Infection by contact

Infection with certain organisms may be acquired via unbroken or broken skin or mucous surfaces by *direct contact* or implantation. This can occur when an infected sore is touched or when an open wound is contaminated directly with soil or dust. In some cases, leptospiral organisms in water seem to be able to penetrate wet skin. Intimate contact, as in kissing, allows infections such as herpes simplex, glandular fever, streptococcal infection and diphtheria to be transmitted. The venereal diseases are transmitted by sexual contact (p.52).

### Infection by ingestion

Some pathogens cause disease when an effective challenge dose has been ingested. The dose of the respective bacteria required to produce bacillary dysentery or typhoid seems to be relatively small, whereas salmonella food poisoning is associated with a high challenge dose (see p.74). The nature of the food or drink may markedly influence the result of the challenge; for example, ingestion of an alkaline drink might interfere with the protective antibacterial action of gastric acid. Water-borne disease is considered in Chapter 9 and food-borne disease in Chapter 10.

### Infection by inhalation

The respiratory avenue of infection is obviously of importance in a wide range of diseases that include many viral, fungal and bacterial infections ranging from the common cold to tuberculosis. Airborne spread of disease is discussed in Chapter 8. Note that infection by an airborne organism may involve a wound, for example, and airborne spread is not restricted to respiratory pathogens.

### Infection by inoculation

The term inoculation was originally used in the botanical sense of implantation of the eye or bud of a plant into a new recipient stock. Infection by inoculation *into* the eye of man, or by implantation on the human conjunctiva, merits consideration in relation to many local and general infections, but this will not be further discussed here. The term inoculation now generally denotes implantation into animal tissues (see note below).

Infection by inoculation may arise in several ways:

(1)    Simply by accidental implantation of an infective agent into or through the skin as a result of a pin prick or thorn prick, by a glass splinter, a stab wound, an injury during sport, a road accident, or a gunshot wound.

(2)    By the use of a contaminated surgical needle or instrument at operations that may range from a needle prick for the preparation of a blood smear to a major operation under anaesthesia.

(3)    By animal bite, or

(4)    By insect bite, as in arthropod-borne diseases (p.82), and in plague (p.81), yellow fever (p.84) and malaria.

### A note on inoculations or injections given in clinical practice

A syringe and needle are frequently used for the *parenteral administration* of various sterile preparations, i.e. administration by a non-intestinal route; the term is used to denote an injection in the usual sense. Different types of injection are recognized according to the level of penetration or the tissue involved (Fig. 6.3).

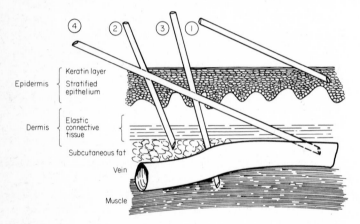

**Figure 6.3**    The structure of skin and an outline of commonly used parenteral routes of injection.

(1)    *Intradermal*
(2)    *Subcutaneous* (or hypodermic)
(3)    *Intramuscular*
(4)    *Intravenous*
(5)    *Intra-arterial*   (not illustrated)

In addition, some special procedures may require the following routes:

intraperitoneal    :    into the peritoneal cavity of the abdomen.
intrathecal    :    into the space near the spinal cord where the cerebrospinal fluid is found.
intracerebral    :    into the brain.
intra-articular    :    into a joint cavity.

## THE SIZE OF THE TRANSMITTED CHALLENGE

The transmission of an infective challenge may be relatively direct from the source to the new host, as in one of the sexually transmitted diseases for example. Here a delicate organism is not normally exposed to the hazards of desiccation or other deleterious influences but is directly implanted on to a susceptible moist epithelial surface in the new host.

Various infections are much less directly transmitted and the source may be more distant from the new host in terms of time and space. The size of the challenge dose transferred is likely to be less as the distance or time from the source is increased, but this in turn depends upon the viability of the organism concerned and innumerable variables that may operate.

In some circumstances, as in a young infants' ward in which gastro-enteritis occurs, one case acts as a source as outlined above but a second and third case in the same ward begins to build up a cumulative threat and the outbreak spreads alarmingly. It might be argued that it is the probability of transmission rather than the size of the transmitted challenge that increases in this situation. Cumulative increases in environmental contamination may similarly occur when a careful check on hygiene is not kept on catering premises or in pig-swill areas near kitchens or in wet areas in ward side-rooms.

The very serious booster effect that occurs when contaminated food is mishandled is discussed later (p.71).

## INFECTIVITY & VIRULENCE

It will now be clear that, in addition to variations in the nature of the attacking organism, there are variables influencing the numbers that may reach the host to deliver a particular challenge at a vulnerable site on or in the host's tissues. This is the critical stage in which the *infectivity* of the pathogen is expressed; it is analogous to the setting up of a bridgehead from which to mount an attack and it involves the breaching of the host defences at some point. The organism then expresses its *virulence*, its capacity to damage or kill the host, by a generalized extension into the host (*invasiveness*) or by the elaboration and release of specific and highly injurious diffusible toxins (*toxigenicity*) or by a combination of these forms of aggression. In most examples of microbial disease in man, these expressions of pathogenicity are associated with successful multiplication of the attacking organism on or in the host (Fig. 6.2).

## PATTERNS OF BACTERIAL ATTACK

It seems that no unitarian hypothesis of microbial pathogenicity is likely to emerge and that each infective syndrome involves its own unique permutation of microbial factors and host responses in its particular host-parasite association. With that important reservation, it is useful to attempt to group bacterial infectious diseases as follows:

(1)    *Localized infection.* Some infections are typically localized in the 'normal'

host; they only occasionally produce widespread effects, although multiple exotoxins and aggressins may be produced. *Staph. aureus* is the classical example of an organism that generally attacks in this way (p.43), and the gonococcus is usually associated with an initially local infection.

(2)  *Localized infection with diffusion of a potent toxin producing a specific 'toxic disease'.* The acute toxic syndromes of diphtheria and tetanus are clear examples (p.44).

(3)  *Local infection with generalized toxin effect ('toxaemia') and bacterial spread.* Streptococcal infections of wounds may extend after the initial establishment of an infective focus. The patient then has fever and feels unwell (malaise) as a result of a non-specific toxaemia.

(4)  *Generalized (invasive) infection.* Some bacteria are from the start typically highly invasive when infection occurs. They sweep through the body, often by blood-borne (haematogenous) spread. They frequently show a predilection for a particular tissue or organ (organotropism) and they may have well recognized portals of entry by which the infective bridgehead was initially achieved. This pattern is seen in some acute bacterial diseases such as plague and typhoid fever and it is also typical of many virus infections (poliomyelitis, smallpox, influenza). Some generalized bacterial infections are recurrent, as in brucellosis (undulant fever), or they may produce a low-grade, progressive disease as in some forms of tuberculosis.

## BACTERIAL ADHESIVENESS

It is becoming clear that many bacteria have an affinity or specific adhesiveness for certain sites on mucosal epithelial surfaces. The diphtheria bacillus localizes in the pharynx, as does the streptococcus that causes acute sore throat. Certain streptococci produce dextran-like substances from sucrose and stick themselves to tooth surfaces, producing the initial step in the development of dental caries. Related streptococci can stick to damaged heart valves. The bacillus that causes whooping cough sticks to the ciliated epithelium of the upper respiratory tract. The cholera vibrio (and probably *Escherichia coli* strains associated with gastro-enteritis in man) can adhere to the epithelial cells of the small intestine.

When pathogens colonize or infect an epithelial surface, they may then cause damage by production of an exotoxin. This is so in the case of diphtheria (p.45), for example. Some pathogens get into the epithelial cells to which they initially attach; they may then kill the cells and cause shallow epithelial ulceration. This is possibly the mechanism of pathogenicity in bacillary dysentery (p.65). Other bacteria seem to penetrate further and multiply in sub-epithelial tissues. They may be taken up by macrophages but, resisting digestion, might even multiply intracellularly. This seems to be the case in the initiation of typhoid fever (p.67).

# TOXIGENICITY

Bacterial products that harm the host have been classified broadly into those secreted from bacterial cells during active growth, the *exotoxins*, and a toxic substance that is an integral part of bacterial cell structure characteristic of Gram-negative bacteria and referred to as *endotoxin*. The classical distinction is indicated in Table 6.1.

The classical exotoxins are potently toxic thermolabile proteins. Each is specific for the particular species; for example, tetanus toxin is produced only by *Clostridium tetani*. Moreover, their toxic activity is directed at specific receptors or systems in the host. Some are known to be lethal in very small amounts. Bacterial toxins are sometimes named in relation to the typical clinical syndrome that they produce (diphtheria toxin, tetanus toxin), but they are generally described in terms of their demonstrable activity in laboratory tests. For example, many bacterial toxins are haemolytic, or leucocidal, or cytolytic. Some are neurotoxins affecting the nervous system, and some are enterotoxins affecting the gut.

**Table 6.1**    Bacterial toxins: The classical concept (now insecure).

| Exotoxins | Endotoxins |
| --- | --- |
| Produced by Gram-positive bacteria | Produced by Gram-negative bacteria |
| Extracellular | Cell-associated |
| Simple protein, thermolabile | Complex lipopolysaccharide, thermostable |
| Very poisonous with high specificity | Moderately so; non-specific* |
| Toxoid stimulates neutralising antitoxin | Not toxoidable; not effectively neutralized |

* Different bacterial endotoxins have individual serological specificity, but their biological toxic effects, which are pharmacologically defined, are shared.

Further work on bacterial toxins has shown that the division into exotoxins and endotoxins was an over-simplification. It is now known that some protein toxins of Gram-negative bacteria are cell-bound or intracytoplasmic. These cannot be termed exotoxins, and they are quite distinct from the classical endotoxin of the cell wall. Moreover, some protein toxins are now known to occur both intracellularly and extracellularly during the active growth phase of certain bacteria. Accordingly, a new classification has been suggested (Table 6.2). True protein exotoxins are sometimes referred to as soluble antigens. They can be rendered non-toxic by treatment with formalin and are then referred to as *toxoids*. A toxoid is usually a good antigen and stimulates the production of antitoxic antibody if injected under suitable conditions into an animal or man.

**Table 6.2**  Classification of bacterial toxins (after Raynaud & Alouf)*.

| |
|---|
| GROUP   I : INTRACYTOPLASMIC PROTEIN TOXINS OF GRAM-NEGATIVE BACTERIA |
| GROUP  II : 'ENDOTOXINS' OF CELL WALLS OF GRAM-NEGATIVE BACTERIA |
| GROUP III : TRUE PROTEIN EXOTOXINS |
| GROUP IV : PROTEIN TOXINS WITH BOTH INTRACELLULAR AND EXTRACELLULAR LOCATION DURING LOG PHASE |

* RAYNAUD M. & ALOUF J.E. (1970) Intracellular versus Extracellular Toxins in *Microbial Toxins* Vol. 1, Chapter 3, p.67—see Suggestions for Further Reading.

## AGGRESSINS

Many bacterial products, whilst not truly toxic in their own right, are likely to enhance the aggressiveness of an organism *in vivo*. Such a substance is hyaluronidase, for example; this breaks down intercellular cement substance and assists the spread of the infecting organism or its products. Other so-called aggressins are proteinase, collagenase, lecithinase (phospholipase), lipase and deoxyribonuclease.

At the present stage of knowledge, we are uncertain of the role of these products in infection and, in some cases, we are not certain that they are invariably produced *in vivo*. Accordingly, Smith has recently pointed out that a toxic or aggressive microbial product can be assigned to one of four categories depending upon its recognized role in the pathogenesis of disease (Table 6.3).

**Table 6.3**  Categories of bacterial toxins in relation to their recognized role in disease (after H. Smith*).

| |
|---|
| (1) ... OF OVER-RIDING IMPORTANCE (e.g. TETANUS TOXIN) |
| (2) ... OF SIGNIFICANCE, BUT NOT THE ONLY FACTOR ... (e.g. 'ENDOTOXIN') |
| (3) ... PRODUCED *IN VITRO*, BUT OF UNKNOWN IMPORTANCE ... (e.g. *SH. SHIGAE* NEUROTOXIN) |
| (4) ... TOXIC EFFECTS *IN VIVO* UNEXPLAINED *IN VITRO* ... (e.g. *STREPT. PNEUMONIAE*) |

* SMITH H. (1968) Biochemical Challenge of Microbial Pathogenicity. *Bacteriological Reviews*, **32**, 164.

This draws attention to our present inability to assess the significance of bacterial endotoxin in disease and to our increasing tendency to consider multifactorial components of disease. These components include microbial and host factors. Current thinking on bacteriogenic shock provides a good example.

## BACTERIOGENIC SHOCK

It has been known for some time that a patient subjected to a release of bacteria or bacterial products into the bloodstream may occasionally become acutely ill with symptoms and signs of shock. The onset is usually sudden; it may be a post-operative event or it may be a sequel to manipulation of an infected area, e.g. catheterization.

The patient may have a rigor (a shivering attack) with fever. The skin may be pale and bluish with the 'cold sweat' of shock and a rapid weak pulse, a falling blood pressure and shallow rapid breathing. Alternatively, but less commonly, the skin is flushed as a result of the release of vasodilatory substances, but the blood pressure is again low; this patient may look misleadingly bright. Thus bacteriogenic shock may insidiously arise to threaten the life of a patient thought to be convalescing uneventfully.

Bacteriogenic shock is typically, but not invariably, associated with bacteriaemic conditions and is sometimes referred to as bacteriaemic shock or septic shock. It is often associated with infections caused by Gram-negative organisms and the synonym 'endotoxic shock' indicates a mechanism that is thought to be involved. However, shock syndromes can also be precipitated by Gram-positive organisms and by organisms that are not strictly bacteria. It is likely that different initiating mechanisms operate in different infections and that there is a fair amount of common ground in the resulting haemodynamic upsets. One of the catastrophes that can occur is a condition known as *disseminated intravascular coagulation* in which, as a consequence of increased capillary permeability and loss of fluid from the vascular system, the blood cells 'sludge' in small vessels and the blood clotting mechanism is activated. This interrupts the blood supply of tissues such as the bowel, the kidney, the lungs and the liver, and scattered areas of cell death (necrosis) are produced. The uncontrolled and generalized clotting uses up the patient's haemostatic (blood coagulating) reserves and there is therefore a tendency to bleed when these foci of damage break down. This calls for prompt and energetic treatment to save the patient from dangerous haemorrhages and, at the same time, to restore the deficient circulation.

## CHANGES IN THE PATHOGEN

### Exaltation and attenuation of virulence

An organism that depends for its virulence on the production of a single toxin becomes avirulent when it mutates to a non-toxigenic variant. Similarly, if an organism's virulence is dependent on its possession of a capsule, as is the case with the pneumococcus, then non-capsulate variants are non-pathogenic; however, this is only so if the capsule plays a primary role in virulence. There are many capsulate organisms that are not virulent for man. The possession of certain superficial somatic chemical groups or antigenic determinants is often of pathogenic significance as these dictate reactions of the organism with host cells and host defence systems. If an organism loses such an antigenic character it may become much less virulent.

When a pathogenic organism multiplies successfully in a susceptible host, it becomes biologically adapted and may well be of enhanced virulence for other susceptible hosts of that species. The virulence of the pathogen can be serially raised or *exalted* by successive transfer ('passage') in this way. On the other hand, successive laboratory subculture of an organism is likely to render it less virulent as it adapts to the artificial environment of culture media and loses the special characters that are selectively advantageous *in vivo*. This is referred to as *attenuation* of virulence in culture and it is of importance in vaccine production as an avirulent organism is likely to have lost antigens that are of significance in its pathogenic role. An antigen concerned in virulence may be rather misleadingly referred to as a protective antigen in this context because the vaccine manufacturer seeks to ensure that his vaccine contains that component in order to stimulate antibodies to it in the vaccinated subject.

### Exotic infections

Infections that are not generally encountered in a country can be imported in various ways, especially as a result of air travel. Accordingly, the clinician is obliged to be alert to an occasional case of a so-called exotic or unusual imported infection occurring in his daily practice. Exotic infections in Britain might include malaria, cholera, smallpox and typhus fever.

## OPPORTUNISTIC PATHOGENS

As the initiation of a disease by any pathogenic organism depends upon innumerable chance happenings, it follows that all pathogens are opportunists. However, the 'opportunistic' label is presently applied to a pathogen that appears to take advantage of unusual circumstances to attack the host; the opportunistic organism is not traditionally associated with the pathogenic role that it adopts, but certain opportunists are already coming to be recognized as having a fairly regular association with certain circumstances. Hence, an aerobic sporeforming organism may be allowed to multiply in a transfusion fluid and may consequently give rise to a clinical catastrophe in a transfused patient, or a relatively benign *Staphylococcus albus* may colonize a man-made heart valve, or a pseudomonas organism may contaminate a metal airway tube and cause an infection in the lungs of a debilitated patient. These events should continue to be unusual; they call for special awareness on the part of the clinical microbiologist who might be tempted to attribute unusual findings to laboratory contamination of his media.

## THE COMPROMISED HOST

Infection is generally more likely to occur in a person whose normal defences are less effective than usual. It is well known, for example, that diabetic patients are more susceptible than healthy subjects to certain infections and that children with immunological deficiencies are particularly vulnerable to certain pathogens (p.31). Similarly, a patient receiving corticosteroid therapy or cytotoxic therapy or immuno-suppressive therapy is compromised in terms of his normal antimicrobial integrity. In consequence, hospital patients include, on the one hand, many people who are at special risk, and on the other hand, many infected patients who are a source of dangerous challenges. These two groups are sometimes linked by hospital personnel or mobile hospital equipment, and aseptic techniques and barrier nursing procedures are designed to ensure that the challenges are not delivered.

## ILLUSTRATIVE EXAMPLES OF BACTERIAL INFECTION

Pathogenic *staphylococci* produce various toxic and aggressive substances and are also responsible for a wide variety of clinical conditions. The commonest are superficial and typically localized boils, styes, carbuncles and abscesses (see p.48). Generalized staphylococcal infections do occur, as in pyaemia (the blood-borne spread of little infected fragments) and bronchopneumonia. The mechanism of pathogenicity of the staphylococcus is not really known. The potentially dangerous staphylococci produce coagulase which has been said to be concerned perhaps in walling off the lesion from host defence mechanisms or may indeed inactivate certain defence mechanisms. The initiation of staphylococcal infection in adult skin is usually associated with a minor wound, a surgical wound—especially if fatty tissue is prominent—a surgical suture (stitch abscess), or a focus of bacterial multiplication in a hair follicle.

The pathogenicity of the *gonococcus* is difficult to explain. This organism appears to be taken into the epithelial lining of the genital tract by a process that partly depends upon the organism's adhesiveness and partly on the phagocytic action of host epithelial cells. At present we know that the gonococcus is pyogenic, but we know very little about its attack mechanisms.

An infection that serves as a model of an acute invasive bacterial attack is lobar pneumonia caused by *Streptococcus pneumoniae* (the *pneumococcus*) (p.61). This is a severe pyrexial illness of sudden onset. The organism is inhaled into the lung tissue, possibly along with some mucus which appears to enhance its initial pathogenicity. There is then progressive invasion of the lung tissue from that infective focus. The pneumococci elicit a host response that includes exudation of fluid and the organisms sweep through the affected lobe, virtually assisted by a wave of exudate that consolidates (literally, renders

43

solid) that section of the lung and puts it out of action. The invasion is only limited by the anatomical boundaries of the lobe, and the multiplying pneumococci often 'spill over' into the general bloodstream so that bacteriaemia occurs.

The virulence of the pneumococcus is related to its possession of a capsule which inhibits normal host phagocytic action; the polymorphs are thereby unable to come to grips with the polysaccharide capsular substance. Within a few days in the surviving patient, however, specific antibodies against the polysaccharide hapten (see p.61) begin to develop and these have an opsonizing effect as they change the surface charge on the capsule. The balance begins to turn in favour of the host, though the large amount of pneumococcal capsular material now present in the lung tissue may initially divert much antibody. In due course, the consolidated lung tissue is resolved and the function of the lobe is restored, but this may take some weeks in the untreated case. Before the advent of effective antimicrobial drugs, lobar pneumonia killed many people.

The pneumococcus produces a haemolysin, a spreading factor (hyaluronidase), and a mucinase (neuraminidase). It does not produce a recognized toxin that we can associate with its high pathogenic potential and, at present, we attribute lobar pneumonia to a series of specific host responses that arise when this respiratory pathogen with the ability to resist phagocytosis sets up a focus of infection in lung tissue.

*Streptococcus pyogenes*, the β-haemolytic streptococcus, causes sore throat and puerperal fever and wound infections and various other diseases (p.49). The organism exists in a variety of groups and types which are antigenically distinct. A major protein antigen of clinical interest is located superficially and is referred to as M protein. This is related to the organism's virulence and protects the streptococcus—not against phagocytosis, but against intracellular digestion once it has been phagocytosed. The streptococcus can therefore survive this component of the host defence system and multiply to produce a veritable battery of toxins and aggressins that can damage the host directly or indirectly. If erythrogenic toxin is produced, scarlet fever may result. If the patient becomes sensitized during a streptococcal infection, rheumatic fever (affecting the joints and heart) or acute nephritis (affecting the kidneys) may occur a few weeks later; these delayed sequelae depend upon special host reactions to the infection.

There are remote parallels here with the pathogenicity of the tubercle bacillus, *Mycobacterium tuberculosis* (p.63). This organism can resist phagocytic digestion because it has a waxy component in its cell wall. The damage that it subsequently produces, for example in lung tissue in adult pulmonary tuberculosis, is a consequence of the tissue reaction in a host who becomes sensitized to the organism.

## ACUTE TOXIC INFECTIONS

In diphtheria and tetanus we have to deal with a single *exotoxin* in each case which seems to be responsible for the clinical signs and symptoms associated with the condition. It is possible that some other factor or factors may be involved in enhancing the accessibility of the particular site of action of the toxin, but we shall here concern ourselves with the main facts.

## Diphtheria

This is a disease characterized by sudden onset of sore throat with exudate, fever and marked toxaemia. The exudate produces a fibrinous layer involving the tonsillar area, sometimes the naso-pharynx, and sometimes the larynx when mechanical obstruction of the airway may occur, especially in small children.

In the local site the organisms multiply and produce potent exotoxin which diffuses widely. It has particular affinity for cardiac muscle, sometimes leading to acute cardiac failure, and for certain nervous tissue.

Much is now known about diphtheria toxin which interferes with a transferase system in host cells and upsets protein synthesis. The production of this toxin by the diphtheria bacillus only occurs when it is lysogenized by (i.e. non-virulently infected with) a particular phage. The diphtheria bacillus is only minimally invasive. It is virulent when it is toxigenic, but it does not typically go on from its local site of infection to produce a generalized bacterial spread. Blood cultures in cases of diphtheria would not ordinarily be positive for the diphtheria bacillus which remains localized at its site of infection, usually in the throat.

If a practitioner is confronted with a case of sore throat which he suspects may be diphtheria, he may take a throat swab for bacteriological confirmation, but it is essential that he should give diphtheria antitoxin to the patient without delay to counteract the toxin which is being produced. He may also give antibiotics. *Prevention* by active immunization is of course the ideal (p.107).

## Tetanus

A similar state of affairs is encountered in *tetanus* which is a dreaded condition produced by an anaerobic spore-forming bacillus *Clostridium tetani* found in the soil, especially in manured soil. This organism produces one of the most potent bacterial toxins known—tetanospasmin.

*Cl. tetani* is not invasive at all and is literally pathogenic by accident. It can exist without causing any harm in the gut of man and animals. It only begins to be of potential danger when it is implanted in the tissues; even then, certain requirements have to be met so that this anaerobe can grow. These predisposing conditions include tissue damage and interference with the normal oxygenation of the area. For example, if washed tetanus spores are inoculated into the limb of an animal, tetanus is not produced, but the condition can be initiated if the inoculation site is subsequently injured sufficiently to allow the organisms to grow locally. When toxin is produced it is absorbed via nervous pathways to the CNS for which it has great affinity. In the spinal cord the toxin interferes with the normal inhibition of the lower motor neurone by the upper motor neurone. This results in hyperexcitability and increased tonus of voluntary

45

muscles with spasms and rigidity. An early sign is spasm of the muscles of the jaw, hence the name 'lockjaw' for tetanus. Once again, antitoxin must be given promptly, but here the affinity of the toxin is so great that it is difficult to undo the union with its receptor in the nervous system. Active immunization against tetanus is discussed later (p.109).

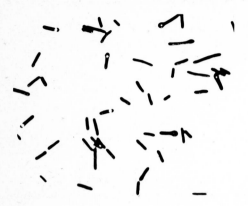

**Plate 1** *Clostridium tetani.*
Smear of a sporing culture. Some of the rod-shaped organisms show sporing forms ranging from darkly staining oval swollen structures (forespores) to terminal round or oval mature spores which do not take up the stain. Methylene blue (X 1080).

# 7 Pyogenic bacteria: wound infections and examples of other common pyogenic infections: examples of bacterial and viral infections acquired by contact or inoculation

The characteristic feature of the host reaction to certain groups of bacteria is the development of pus—the *pyogenic response* (p.28). Bacteria provoking such a reaction are referred to as the pyogenic bacteria and they include some of the pathogenic Gram-negative bacilli and both Gram-positive and Gram-negative cocci. It does not follow that other bacteria are not from time to time associated with pus production. The appearance of the pus varies depending on the organism involved. Staphylococci produce rather thick white or cream-coloured pus, whereas streptococcal pus is typically straw-coloured and fluid; these appearances are often encountered in clinical work, but they are not invariably indicative of the organism.

In accounts of the development of surgery in previous centuries, the term 'laudable pus' was used, presumably because a surgeon was happy to find pus as an indication that he had correctly guessed the site of his patient's trouble. Moreover, in deep-seated infections the release of pus is often associated with improvement in the patient's condition, provided that the primary infection is controlled, and the production of pus is at least an indication of an active host response to a pathogen.

Pus is not invariably produced as a frankly septic exudate. It may be evident microscopically in the urine or in the cerebrospinal fluid; after centrifugation of such a specimen to collect its cellular content, a smear of the deposit may be prepared for microscopical examination in the laboratory and a sample of the deposit may be cultured to detect the pathogen.

In theory, the common infections caused by the various pyogenic bacteria should now be controlled by modern antimicrobial agents. In practice, you will find that the pyogenic cocci are a constant cause of trouble giving rise to much morbidity and a considerable number of deaths. They cause trouble in very many ways and are involved in infections following accidental wounds, post-operative wound infections, and various common infective conditions associated with the skin, throat (tonsillitis, pharyngitis), ears (otitis), eyes (conjunctivitis), sinuses (sinusitis), and other systems. The pyogenic bacilli are also involved in some of these sites and are also a regular cause of primary infections of the urinary tract.

Accordingly, it is necessary to know something of the systematic bacteriology of these pyogenic organisms.

The STAPHYLOCOCCI are Gram-positive cocci that typically occur in clusters. They can be simply classified into three broad categories on the basis of their pigment production on certain media: *Staphylococcus aureus*, producing golden colonies; *Staph. albus*, white colonies; and other pigmented strains such as *Staph. citreus* etc., producing various other colours from lemon-yellow to orange. As non-pigmented variants of *Staph. aureus* produce white colonies, the simple classification is not entirely reliable. Typical *Staph. aureus* strains produce an enzyme 'coagulase' that activates a clotting system in citrated human or rabbit plasma. Coagulase activity is generally associated with pathogenic potential in staphylococci and, for convenience, coagulase-positive staphylococci tend to be labelled *Staph. aureus* or *Staph. pyogenes aureus*. Coagulase-negative, normally non-pathogenic staphylococci, are labelled *Staph. albus* or *Staph. epidermidis albus* as they abound as commensals on the skin. Occasionally, *Staph. albus* causes infection when special circumstances allow, such as the implantation of artificial valves in some patients.

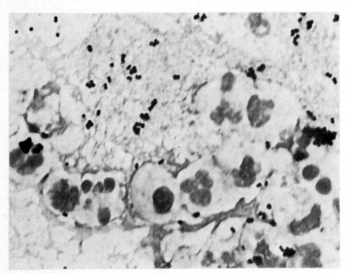

**Plate 2** *Staphylococcal pus.*
The small darkly staining cocci are arranged singly, sometimes in pairs, and typically in small clumps. Degenerate nuclei of pus cells are seen, and there is a background of amorphous material. Gram stain (X 1080).

Staphylococci occur as commensals just within the nostrils (anterior nares) and a significant proportion of the general population carry strains of *Staph. aureus* there (20-30%). Nasal carriers of pathogenic staphylococci are more

48

common among hospital personnel and long-term patients as the hospital environment favours the selection of pathogenic strains. Some people carry staphylococci in other sites, such as the perineum.

*Staphylococcus aureus* is the causative organism of boils, styes and carbuncles, various skin infections such as impetigo and pemphigus (an infection of newborn children) and wound infections. The organism is also a common cause of breast abscess in the nursing mother and osteomyelitis, a localized infection caused by lodgement of blood-borne staphylococci in the small vessels of a long bone.

*Staph. aureus* produces various toxins and aggressins. Some strains produce an enterotoxin that causes food poisoning (p.76).

Some staphylococci encountered in the general population are sensitive to penicillin, but many of the strains found in hospital personnel and acquired by in-patients are resistant to penicillin. These resistant strains destroy penicillin by producing penicillinase, a $\beta$-lactamase, and this gives them a survival advantage in hospitals (pp.97, 104). Staphylococci are often resistant to a variety of antimicrobial drugs; in some cases multiple resistance is conferred by the acquisition of an R-factor as a result of transduction by a phage.

Staphylococci are susceptible to the action of various phages (bacterial viruses) that have specific affinity for them. Accordingly, 'phage types' of staphylococci can be distinguished on the basis of their patterns of sensitivity or resistance to the lytic effects of a series of phages. This is the basis of a system of phage typing that is of epidemiological value.

STREPTOCOCCI are Gram-positive cocci that occur typically in chains. They can be classified on an elementary basis according to the effects produced by their colonies on horse blood agar. Colonies of *Streptococcus pyogenes* are surrounded by zones of clear haemolysis termed *beta*-haemolysis. *Strept. viridans* colonies produce zones of greenish discolouration—*alpha*-haemolysis. *Strept. faecalis* usually produces no haemolysis and, unlike the others, is able to grow on bile-containing media such as MacConkey medium.

*Streptococcus pyogenes* may be carried in the throat of 10-20% of the apparently healthy population; nasal carriers also occur. The organism is typically associated with acute sore throat with exudate (follicular tonsillitis). It can also cause infection of the middle ear (otitis media), skin infections (erysipelas and impetigo), and infections of wounds and burns. These strepto-cocci produce various cytolytic toxins including haemolysins, and various other aggressins. They cause scarlet fever by producing erythrogenic toxin; scarlet fever is really a tonsillitis infection with an accompanying rash. In some cases, an infection with *Strept. pyogenes* is followed several weeks later by rheumatic fever or acute glomerulonephritis. These are serious hypersen-sitivity reactions affecting the kidneys in glomerulonephritis and the joints and the heart in the case of rheumatic fever.

Strains of *Streptococcus pyogenes* can be sub-grouped into Lancefield's groups A—S on the basis of precipitation reactions that depend upon the presence of a group-specific carbohydrate (C antigen) at the surface of the

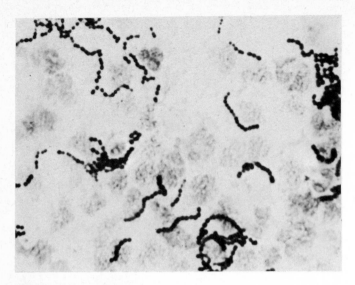

**Plate 3**  *Streptococcal pus.*
The cocci are arranged in chains against a background of cell debris. The pus cells have been typically decomposed by the products of the streptococci. Gram stain (X 1080).

streptococcus. The most important group is Group A in terms of pathogenic associations with man. As Group A streptococci are typically sensitive to bacitracin, a bacitracin-sensitivity test is often used to provide presumptive evidence of the group. Bacitracin is not often used therapeutically because it is potentially toxic. The drug of choice for the treatment of infections caused by *Strept. pyogenes* is penicillin. This organism is invariably sensitive to penicillin whereas resistance to tetracycline is not uncommon.

The *Strept. viridans* group abound as commensals in the mouth and oro-pharynx. These organisms may be associated with dental disease. Related streptococci (*Strept. mutans, Strept. sanguis* etc.) can produce dextran-like substances from sucrose and stick themselves to tooth surfaces. This is the mechanism of the formation of dental plaque—a film of polysaccharide material associated with the development of dental caries and periodontal disease. Viridans streptococci are very numerous in the mouth and may occasionally gain access to the blood stream; if a person has a congenital heart disorder or has damaged heart valves as a result of previous rheumatic fever, *Strept. viridans* in the blood may alight on these damaged areas and cause a condition termed *subacute bacterial endocarditis*. Streptococci of the viridans group are usually sensitive to penicillin.

The *Strept. faecalis* group are commensals of the gut and are sometimes referred to as the enterococci. They can cause infections of abdominal wounds and they are often found, along with *Escherichia coli*, in association with infections of the urinary tract. *Strept. faecalis* organisms are usually resistant to penicillin.

*Streptococcus pneumoniae*, the pneumococcus, is described in a later chapter (p.61).

*ESCHERICHIA COLI* is a Gram-negative rod-shaped organism. It occurs as a commensal in the gut of man and animals and its presence in water supplies is regarded as an index of faecal contamination. Many organisms abound in nature that are similar to *Esch. coli*, but these are sometimes saprophytic and they are not necessarily derived from faeces. For this reason, the identification of 'typical *Esch. coli*' has special significance (p.70).

*Esch. coli* and related organisms that may occur in the gut of man are frequently involved in infections of the urinary tract. The usual route of invasion is generally assumed to be by retrograde spread up the urethra to the bladder to produce cystitis and thence via the ureters to the kidneys to produce pyelonephritis. These infections are particularly common in women of child-bearing age.

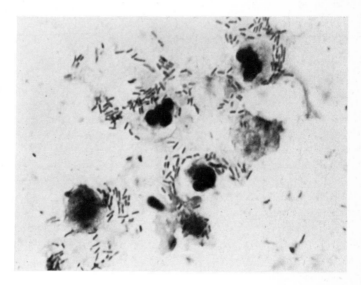

**Plate 4**    *Escherichia coli* pus.
Many rod-shaped bacteria are present with pus cells and debris. Gram stain (X 1080).

Although the commensal role of *Esch. coli* in the gut is well recognized, certain strains called 'enteropathogenic *Esch. coli*' are associated with severe gastro-enteritis of infants. Outbreaks of this form of gastro-enteritis in neonatal units are very dangerous and tend to spread rapidly. In general, *Esch. coli* may be fiercely invasive in the neonate and it is a common cause of neonatal septicaemia and meningitis. Strains of *Esch. coli* are also thought to be associated with diarrhoeal disease in adults, especially traveller's diarrhoea in which it is assumed that the newcomer is challenged by a strain that he has not previously encountered.

*Esch. coli*, alone or in combination with other faecal organisms, may be involved in abdominal or pelvic infections. Post-operative complications such as

51

stitch abscess, wound sepsis or peritonitis may be caused by *Esch. coli*. The organism is typically penicillin-resistant and it is often resistant to various other antibiotics.

*Esch. coli* is the Pandora's box of the microbial geneticists in that it has afforded much insight into mechanisms of wide biological interest and it also has a great capacity for harm. The process of conjugation and transfer of bits of DNA (plasmids) conferring various properties including multiple drug resistance is of special medical interest (p.104).

## AN EXAMPLE OF EXOGENOUS INFECTION ACQUIRED BY DIRECT CONTACT: THE VENEREAL DISEASES

The venereal diseases are so called because they are typically transmitted by intimate sexual contact. As the term venereal denotes loving and as transmission of such infection may involve a degree of thoughtlessness or a casual encounter, it is now considered more reasonable to refer to this group of infections as 'sexually acquired diseases'. Our fashionably permissive society is faced with the third major epidemic of gonorrhoea in the present century and this time without war-induced dislocations of population to account for the situation. Now that birth control is more effectively available in pill form to large numbers of young women, and with the lack of a degree of protection that can be afforded by the male use of a sheath, the increased transmission of gonorrhoea reflects our changing habits and practices.

The most common venereal disease is gonorrhoea caused by *Neisseria gonorrhoeae*, the gonococcus, which is a pyogenic organism. Syphilis, nowadays much less common than formerly, is caused by a spirochaete, *Treponema pallidum*, which is not pyogenic. Apart from the mode of their transmission, these diseases and their causative organisms have virtually nothing in common, but it is significant that both of the organisms seem to be very delicate and their infectivity is lost quickly if they are not protected and directly implanted on a favourable site in the new host. The gonococcus and the spirochaete are highly species-specific and, as they do not readily produce any disease in animals, research into their pathogenicity has been hampered. The source of infection in each case is another human being. With a few exceptions such as congenitally acquired syphilis or infection of a baby's eyes with gonorrhoea at birth, the primary site involved is usually the genitalia and sometimes the rectum or mouth.

The gonococcus can be cultured on specially enriched media; its successful isolation in the laboratory demands care and attention to detail including incubation with added carbon dioxide.

Some workers have claimed that they have cultured *Treponema pallidum*, but it is generally held that it is not yet possible to culture this organism. Accordingly, the diagnosis of syphilis often rests upon indirect serological evidence unless the organism has been identified with reasonable confidence in the early stages of the disease when it may be visualized by special microscopical methods.

52

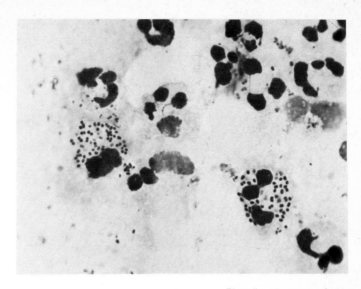

**Plate 5** *Gonococcal pus.*
The small darkly staining diplococci are typically seen within polymorphs (pus cells). The boundaries of the pus cells are indistinct and some of these cells are breaking up. The polymorph nuclei are clearly evident. Modified Gram stain (X 1080).

## AN ILLUSTRATIVE ENDOGENOUS INFECTION: URINARY TRACT IN-FECTION

Urine is a good culture medium for many bacterial species, including the coliform bacteria and enterococci that abound in the human colon. The maintenance of the sterility of the urinary tract depends upon various anti-bacterial mechanisms, and the efficiency of the system in dealing with retrograde spread of organisms from the regularly contaminated perineal area is markedly compromised by anything that interferes with the hydrodynamics of the flushing system. Moreover, if the bladder is not completely emptied and a significant amount of residual urine remains, there is the possibility that a continuous culture system can be set up.

The relative shortness of the female urethra and its anatomical location render it more vulnerable than the male urethra to the implantation of endogenous potentially pathogenic organisms and to local trauma that might assist retrograde infection.

It is therefore easy to understand why *Escherichia coli* and related bacteria, *Proteus mirabilis, Pseudomonas aeruginosa,* and *Streptococcus faecalis,* are commonly encountered as urinary tract pathogens (Table 7.1), and why infections of the urinary tract are common in women, especially in women of child-bearing age, in whom the local trauma of sexual intercourse and the various changes associated with pregnancy are recognized as contributory factors. Urinary tract infection is also common in children who have congenital malformations of the urinary tract, and it is well recognized as a complication of prostatic trouble in older men.

53

**Table 7.1**  The relative occurrence of bacteria associated with urinary tract infections.

| | Percentage | Occurrence |
|---|---|---|
| | in 17,411 in-patients | in 6,080 out-patients |
| *Escherichia coli* | 47 | 64 |
| *Proteus mirabilis* | 21 | 15 |
| *Klebsiella aerogenes* | 7 | 4 |
| Coliform bacteria | 17 | 9 |
| Gram-positive bacteria | 8 | 8 |

From MCALLISTER T.A., ALEXANDER J.G., DULAKE C., PERCIVAL A., BOYCE J.M.H. & WORMALD P.J. (1971) Multicentric study of sensitivities of urinary tract pathogens. *Postgraduate Medical Journal* (September Suppl. 1971) 47, 7–14.

The laboratory diagnosis of urinary tract infection presents problems because urine is readily contaminated during urination, and bacteria can multiply readily in the warm specimen before it is examined at the laboratory. There are several solutions to each of the problems; one approach is as follows:

(1)   A 'mid-stream' or 'clean-catch' specimen of urine is taken and examined promptly, or it is promptly chilled and held cold until it is examined. Especially in the case of female patients it is essential to take special steps to avoid contamination at this stage.

(2)   The deposit obtained from a centrifuged sample is examined microscopically for pus cells and bacteria. Red blood cells and epithelial cells may also be present.

(3)   A sample of the uncentrifuged urine is serially diluted and a viable count (colony count) is performed by culturing standard volumes (drops or pipetted amounts) of each dilution on plates of nutrient medium. Acceptable 'short-cut' procedures are available. It is then possible to calculate the number of viable organisms per ml of urine.

The occurrence of bacteria in the urine ('bacteriuria') is often attributable to simple external contamination of the specimen. This is particularly likely to be so if there are relatively small numbers of organisms and a relatively large variety of different species representing the varied commensal and transient flora of the perineum. So-called *'significant bacteriuria'*, i.e. indicating the likelihood of a true infection, is associated with relatively large numbers of bacteria belonging to one or two (less commonly more than two) species.

The laboratory guideline, provided that the specimen has been taken and submitted properly is:

> Viable count less than $10^4$ organisms per ml   = contamination
> Viable count more than $10^5$ organisms per ml = significant bacteriuria
> A count between $10^4$ and $10^5$ calls for a repeat investigation.

These guidelines must, of course, be considered together with clinical details and the result of microscopy etc., in assessing an individual case.

# A LIFE-THREATENING PYOGENIC INFECTION

## Acute (purulent) bacterial meningitis

Acute bacterial infections of the membranes that surround the brain and spinal cord (meningitis) arise when certain bacteria gain access to the cerebro-spinal system from the blood stream or via peri-neural lymphatic channels accompanying the olfactory nerve from the area of the nasal sinuses into the skull. The organisms multiply in the cerebro-spinal fluid (CSF) which can be sampled for laboratory investigation by an aseptic procedure known as *lumbar puncture*.

The bacteria most commonly associated with acute meningitis are indicated in Table 7.2. As these organisms have inherently different antibiotic sensitivities,

Table 7.2    The major causes of bacterial meningitis reported in Scotland 1970—74.

| Causative organism | Number of cases |
|---|---|
| *Neisseria meningitidis* | 281 |
| *Haemophilus* spp. | 169 |
| *Strept. pneumoniae* | 149 |
| Staphylococci | 68 |
| Coliform organisms* | 60 |
| Streptococci (excl. pneumococci) | 54 |
| *M. tuberculosis* | 16 |

* Other cases were caused by *Proteus, Klebsiella, Pseudomonas, Salmonella* and *Achromobacter* spp. Data for Tables 7.2 and 7.3 from Communicable Diseases (Scotland) (CDS) Reports.

and as strains also vary in their particular sensitivities, it is most important to identify the organisms and to monitor therapy with antibiotic sensitivity tests. Table 7.3 shows that viruses accounted for a number of cases with meningitic reactions in the two years 1972—73 comparable with those caused by bacteria in the five years 1970—74 in Scotland. This illustrates a further problem in diagnosis; whereas the treatment of viral meningitis is largely supportive, the treatment of bacterial meningitis is undeniably therapeutic and these cases must not be missed. Investigations of clinical interest include

Table 7.3    The major causes of viral meningitis and/or encephalitis reported in Scotland in 1972—73.

| Virus | Number of cases |
|---|---|
| Echovirus | 282 |
| Mumps | 191 |
| Coxsackie Virus | 65 |
| Herpes Simplex Virus | 40 |
| Adenovirus | 23 |
| Influenza | 17 |
| Measles | 17 |

microscopy of a centrifuged deposit to determine the bacterial content and the host cell response; the presence of pus cells indicates an acute bacterial infection. Culture of the deposit may yield the causative organism. The chemistry of the CSF is also of interest. In a typical acute bacterial infection, the protein content of the fluid is increased, and the glucose content is markedly decreased.

## EXAMPLES OF VIRUS DISEASES ACQUIRED BY CONTACT OR INOCULATION

### Herpes simplex

Herpes simplex virus (*herpesvirus hominis*) is typically associated with vesicular 'cold sores' that occur on the lips. These are usually recurrent infections; it seems that, after a primary infection which often occurs in childhood, the virus produces a latent infection in the area or in the nerve supply of the area and is activated from time to time by stimuli such as strong sunlight or local heat or a fevered state. The resulting sore sheds infectious virus.

The virus occurs in two antigenic types (1 and 2). Type 1 is usually associated with facial infections and type-2 strains are associated with genital infections (though type 1 can occur here also). Genital herpes in adults is now regarded as a venereal disease, and herpes simplex generally is an example of a virus that is transmitted by close contact or by mediate contact with heavily contaminated articles such as shared cups.

Laboratory diagnosis of *herpesvirus hominis* rests upon the growth of the organism in a cell culture and the production of a cytopathic effect which can be inhibited by antiserum. Complement-fixation tests and neutralization tests provide serological evidence that can be useful but may be confusing in cases of recurrent infection which are not accompanied by typical antibody responses. The reason for this is not clear.

Herpes simplex virus is in the same group as the virus of herpes zoster and chicken pox (varicella-zoster virus), but it is quite distinct from that virus.

### Viral hepatitis B (serum hepatitis)

This is a worrying form of infectious jaundice usually acquired by accidental injury under circumstances that allow at least traces of human blood from a case or carrier to gain access to the tissues of the new host. The incubation period is typically long (50-150 days) and the infection varies in severity from clinically inapparent to fulminating and fatal hepatitis.

There is little doubt that the virus has been visualized; three forms are demonstrable by electron microscopy ranging from a small (core) particle of 18-22 nm to the so-called Dane particle that has outer and inner membranes around the icosahedral core and looks like a virus. A specific antigen, called Australia (Au) antigen because it was originally detected in an aborigine, can be demonstrated by various procedures including immunodiffusion, immuno-electrophoresis and radio-immunoassay.

56

It seems that the carrier state is influenced by immune deficiencies and that the actual disease is precipitated by immune complex mechanisms in the patient; there appears to be a measure of immunosuppression during the illness.

Hepatitis B is a recognized occupational hazard for those who may come into contact with human blood or serum; careful precautions must be taken by surgeons, nurses, pathologists, para-clinical technicians and laboratory workers. There is early evidence that venereal transmission of this agent is of significance.

# 8 Respiratory transmission and airborne infection

Our normal behaviour reflects our awareness of the respiratory avenue of infection and the airborne spread of disease. We intuitively endeavour to keep at a distance from a visitor who has a cold, and we do not exchange kisses with a member of the family who has an infection involving the respiratory tract or oro-pharynx. We recoil from a child with the whoop of whooping-cough and we nurse patients with pulmonary tuberculosis in well-ventilated rooms. However, associated with each of these examples are areas of considerable doubt regarding exact pathways and mechanisms of airborne infection.

Examples of virus diseases that may be spread by the respiratory route include coryza (the common cold), influenza, measles and smallpox. The classical bacterial examples include pulmonary tuberculosis and lobar pneumonia. The mycoplasmas, *Coxiella burnetii* and the fungi are also well represented among the pathogens spread by airborne routes.

When a person coughs or sneezes or spits, a *droplet spray* of small and large droplets is expelled. This may transfer certain infections. The larger droplets do not travel far but may contaminate clothing, or flooring, or nearby inanimate objects within a few feet of their source and they add their infective contribution to dust; subsequently, air currents may carry *dust-borne particles* that can be inhaled. If organisms are not exposed to ultraviolet light or strong direct sunlight under these latter conditions, some—such as smallpox virus, tubercle bacilli, staphylococci and streptococci—can survive the degree of desiccation that is involved and remain infective for days or weeks. Thus a school teacher with an undiagnosed cough or a patient with a discharging wound may contaminate their surroundings or their contacts in dangerous ways.

In addition, fine droplets evaporate rapidly in transit and these then form *droplet nuclei*; some of these may carry infecting organisms and can be inhaled directly. However, droplet spray and droplet nuclei are not generally regarded as being such a potent source of trouble as infected dust. This concept might be challenged in relation to the early infective stage of some virus infections such as measles and smallpox, for example, and recent evidence suggests that the saliva may be more directly dangerous in cases of streptococcal infection, but the generally held view is that the microbial pathogens in actual infected secretions from the nose, throat and chest are less significantly transmitted in droplet sprays and are more effectively distributed as follows:

*Nasal exudate* contaminates hands and handkerchiefs and clothing.

*Throat secretions* and *sputum* may be coughed or spat directly on to handkerchiefs, clothing, furniture or floor. (It is important to visualize these unpleasant occurrences in the microscopic as well as the macroscopic sense).

The hands of a person during normal conversation regularly touch his or her face and nose and may transfer organisms such as nasal staphylococci or streptococci directly or indirectly to other people. Opportunities for direct transfer are greatest at times of close contact as in kissing, and indirect transfer might be quite efficient if a common cup is shared, or if children put a shared pencil or toy in their mouths, or if a mother uses her handkerchief to 'clean' the child's nose, lip or eye. The handkerchief is a formidable store of danger under these circumstances and it is surprising that the custom of retaining such a dirty item about our person persists in this age of disposables. The pathways of potential infection discussed here (see Fig. 8.1) are fairly evident, but they

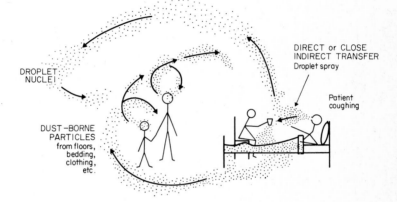

**Figure 8.1**   Visiting challenges.

include varying degrees of direct or indirect transfer and they also include routes that may be classified under respiratory infection, oro-pharyngeal infection, contact infection, or even infection by the conjunctival route.

### The hazard of infected dust

The risk of dust-borne spread of infection is increased when people move together in poorly ventilated conditions, when a handkerchief is waved about, when contaminated clothing is moved by normal body movements or during dressing or undressing, by bed-making, and by dry dusting procedures.

## EXAMPLES OF THE RESPIRATORY ROUTE OF INFECTION

Certain generalized infections that affect superficial cells may also involve cells on mucosal surfaces and, quite early in the disease, the infectious agent may be shed from mucosal surfaces and occur in their related secretions in large numbers. This is true of measles and smallpox and various other diseases. It seems that the measles virus is readily inactivated or diluted to less than an infective challenge unless it is transferred directly to a susceptible new host across relatively small distances. For example, when a family doctor returns home to his own family after seeing young children involved in a measles epidemic, he does not transmit the disease to his own young children or to his wife. His clothes and possibly his face and hands (if he has not washed very thoroughly) may well carry measles virus. He and his wife will normally be immune, having had measles in childhood. His youngest child of 3 months may retain a degree of passively acquired maternal antibody; but his older children of 2 and 4 years may be highly susceptible, unless they were vaccinated against measles (p.109). The fact is that these children do not acquire an infective dose of measles virus from their father. However, the first one to be challenged in the course of close contact with a developing case of measles in one of their young friends, often at nursery school, will bring the infection home. Then the measles virus is transmitted in a significantly effective dose to the other non-immune members of the family. The youngest may still avoid the infection on account of his waning but still protective maternal antibody, but the two-year-old is likely to develop measles (see Fig. 8.2).

With the more resistant, more highly infective smallpox virus, the situation is entirely different. The amount of infective virus that may be transmitted via

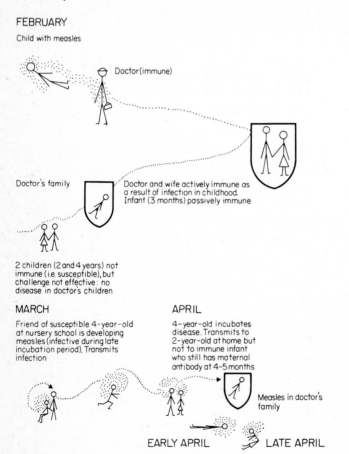

FEBRUARY

Child with measles

Doctor (immune)

Doctor's family

Doctor and wife actively immune as a result of infection in childhood. Infant (3 months) passively immune

2 children (2 and 4 years) not immune (i.e. susceptible), but challenge not effective: no disease in doctor's children

MARCH

Friend of susceptible 4-year-old at nursery school is developing measles (infective during late incubation period). Transmits infection

APRIL

4-year-old incubates disease. Transmits to 2-year-old at home but not to immune infant who still has maternal antibody at 4-5 months

Measles in doctor's family

EARLY APRIL        LATE APRIL

**Figure 8.2** The typical epidemiology of measles in an unvaccinated family.

60

clothing can be dangerous. Under the circumstances described above for measles, the whole family would be at serious risk in the case of smallpox; accordingly, any doctor dealing with a suspected case of smallpox must take special precautions to avoid transmitting the disease.

In the case of pneumococcal pneumonia, the situation is again different. It seems that a virulent strain of the organism may spread in a community at the sub-clinical carrier level. The organism then colonizes the upper respiratory tract and, when suitable atmospheric conditions combine with lowered host resistance and various other factors in individual cases, the pneumococcus may become invasive in the lower respiratory tract (p.43).

### General Precautions

Some of the general precautions that should be taken to avoid airborne infection will be self-evident from the above considerations. Other general precautions include the isolation of cases; the provision of adequate ventilation— in schools, offices, places of entertainment, in buses and trains, and in hospitals—to avoid a build-up of infective challenges; and the avoidance of undue movement of people and of bed linen in hospital wards. It is good practice to restrict attention to wounds in wards to times when airborne organisms are likely to be at minimum rather than maximum numbers, and it might well be argued that dressings should not be changed in the general ward.

These latter considerations move our discussion from the area of respiratory infection to airborne infection of wounds (see p.88).

### Special Hazards

Laboratory workers recognize the danger of inhalation of aerosols that can be produced by simple manipulation of fluids containing pathogens. For example, infective sprays of organisms may arise when specimen bottles or tubes are uncapped or when suspensions are pipetted or centrifuged or handled in a syringe (p.112). Dangerous pathogens should be handled in a suitable protective cabinet so that these risks are minimized. In some cases, masks and protective eye shields should be worn and special consideration should be given to effective ventilation or the use of laminar airflow (see Figs. 8.3, 8.4, 8.5).

### STREPTOCOCCUS PNEUMONIAE

This organism, referred to as the pneumococcus because of its association with lobar pneumonia, typically occurs in pairs as 'lanceolate diplococci', i.e. two slightly ovoid Gram-positive cocci each having a pointed end but apposed at their blunt ends. *Strept. pneumoniae* occurs as a commensal of the upper respiratory tract and, as a pathogen, primarily in the respiratory tract or in related sites such as the sinuses, middle ear, eye or cerebrospinal system.

The organism causes lobar pneumonia, bronchopneumonia, sinusitis, otitis media, conjunctivitis and meningitis. When it is virulent it has a polysaccharide capsule that acts as a hapten (an incomplete antigen) and allows serological sub-

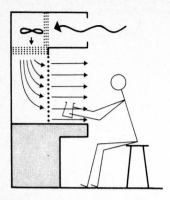

**Figure 8.3** 'Protective cabinet A': With a system of this type, filtered air passes across materials that are thus protected from airborne contamination. Infective material must not be handled in such a cabinet, because the airstream is directed at the operator. This system protects the work, not the worker.

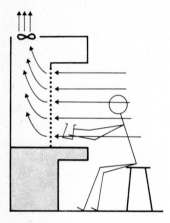

**Figure 8.4** 'Protective cabinet B': With this system, unfiltered (contaminated) air is drawn past the operator and across the working area. The operator is protected to some extent from airborne infection derived from the work in hand. Care must be taken in dealing with the airstream discharged at the top of the system. This system may protect the worker, but it may compromise the work and it may seriously challenge others if its discharge is not considered.

classification of strains into various types. This can be done by an agglutination test or by the capsule-swelling reaction; the specific capsular substance reacts with homologous antiserum and appears to swell when viewed with the microscope. Capsulate pneumococci produce smooth shiny colonies, whereas non-capsulate strains produce matt rough colonies (S-R variation). Thus, virulence in pneumococci is directly related to possession of a capsule (see p.44) and this is linked with type-specificity and the smooth colony form.

Young colonies of *Strept. pneumoniae* resemble those of *Strept. viridans*, but older colonies of pneumococci develop flat tops, often with concentric

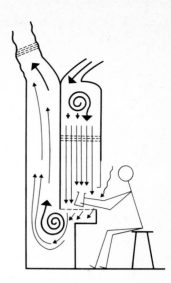

**Figure 8.5** 'Protective cabinet C': Here, a laminar flow of filtered air travels downwards across the work in the cabinet. A small amount of unfiltered air may be 'bled in' past the operator, but not on to the work. The spent air is discharged with safety precautions, sometimes involving a heat-sterilizing system or special filters. In suitable cases, some of the discharged air is recycled through the input filters again.

valleys and ridges. This is the classical 'draughtsman' appearance. The solubility of pneumococci in bile, their sensitivity to the chemical optochin, and the marked virulence of capsulate strains for mice further distingusihes them.

*Strept. pneumoniae* is invariably sensitive to penicillin and often sensitive to sulphonamides or tetracycline.

## MYCOBACTERIUM TUBERCULOSIS

This slender rod-shaped bacillus has waxy (mycolic acid) constituents in its cell wall. When a red dye is driven into the organism by a mordanting procedure in which the stain is heated (the Ziehl-Neelsen method), the stained bacillus then resists the effects of acid treatment or alcohol treatment which readily decolourize other organisms stained in this way. The tubercle bacillus is therefore referred to as 'acid-and-alcohol fast', and the acid-fast characteristic is shared in varying degree by other mycobacteria (including the leprosy bacillus).

*M. tuberculosis* grows much less rapidly than other common pathogens and special media are required. On Lowenstein-Jensen medium, which is commonly used, colonies develop after about 2—3 weeks or more at 37°C. The cultures are grown on solid media cast in small bottles containing enough air for this obligate aerobe but fitted with a screw-cap so that moisture is retained and the dangerous organisms are sealed in. The tubercle bacillus can survive desiccation and can remain viable for weeks or months in dust. The organism is readily

63

inactivated by heat and killed by pasteurization; this is of great importance in relation to the routine treatment of milk (see below).

*Mycobacterium bovis* is the bovine type of tubercle bacillus that occurs in cattle and may contaminate milk. It is not characteristically associated with human pulmonary tuberculosis because the alimentary avenue of infection is more likely to be involved in this case and abdominal tuberculosis or tuberculosis of lymph nodes, bones and joints may result if unpasteurized infected milk is taken. The vaccine used for the prevention of tuberculosis in man (bacille Calmette et Guérin; BCG) is derived from *M. bovis* grown under attenuating conditions so that its virulence for man is reduced; the bovine tubercle bacillus is so closely related to the human type that cross-immunity is conferred by the living vaccine.

The bacteriological diagnosis of tuberculosis rests upon the detection of the acid-fast bacillus in specimens such as sputum which may be specially treated before microscopic examination. The material is also cultured and, in certain cases, test inoculation of a guinea-pig may be necessary to isolate the organism.

## THE INFLUENZA VIRUS

The flu virus is one of the myxoviruses and has affinity for specific mucoid substrates that occur at or in cell surfaces. There are three types of flu virus (A, B, C), of which type C is the most benign and types A and B have epidemic potential. The type-B virus is relatively stable in its antigenic structure which exhibits 'antigenic drift' through the years, whereas type A is notoriously able to change gear from 'antigenic drift' to marked antigenic change from time to time. This can occur at intervals of many years; the changed virus then has the ability to spread widely in hosts who have no immunity to it, and epidemics and pandemics of flu then occur.

Flu is characterized by fever and headache of fairly sudden onset with muscle aches and upper respiratory symptoms. The illness lasts for 3-5 days but respiratory complications are common and bronchopneumonia or an exacerbation of chronic bronchitis often arises in older patients. The bacterium *Haemophilus influenzae* is commonly associated with these secondary infections and was mistakenly labelled as the primary pathogen of flu. The flu virus can be cultured from the throat of patients during the acute phase if material is inoculated into fertile hen eggs, and serological evidence of the disease is readily obtained by complement-fixation or haemagglutination-inhibition rests (pp.12, 14). The latter test exploits the haemagglutinating activity of the flu virus in which it exhibits its affinity for mucoprotein receptors on red cells and sticks the cells together.

# 9 Diseases acquired by ingestion

## I. HAND-TO-MOUTH INFECTION: BACILLARY DYSENTERY

Bacillary dysentery is a diarrhoeal illness caused by the *Shigella* group of Gram-negative rod-shaped bacteria. It is quite distinct from amoebic dysentery which is caused by *Entamoeba histolytica*; the latter is not discussed in this chapter. The most common cause of bacillary dysentery in Britain is *Shigella sonnei*, but some cases are caused by *Sh. flexneri*. *Sh. dysenteriae* and *Sh. boydii* are generally associated with more severe illness and are rarely encountered here. In Britain, the disease is thought to be transmitted by the hand-to-mouth route and it is significant that it primarily spreads among groups who are not able to cope effectively with diarrhoeal problems. Thus, young primary school-children and children at day nurseries are often infected and the infection is most likely to be acquired in or near a communal lavatory (Fig. 9.1). The infection may then spread to the mothers who attend to the

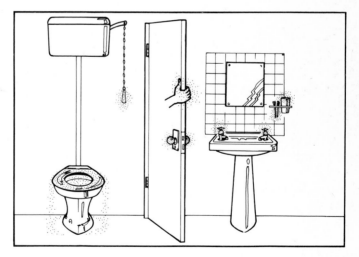

**Figure 9.1** Bacillary dysentery is a recognized hand-to-mouth infection (and indirectly a handle-to-mouth hazard).

infected children. Further spread within an affected household is common. Bacillary dysentery used to be called asylum dysentery as it was recognized that the disease spread readily among those who could not observe simple rules of personal hygiene.

Shigella infections are essentially specific for man. Bacillary dysentery involves the large bowel and there is inflammation of the mucosa, sometimes leading to extensive superficial ulceration with sloughing. The clinical picture is variable. The disease usually presents as acute diarrhoea lasting for several days. The diarrhoea may be profuse and frequent, with frank blood and pus in the stools, but in some cases it is quite mild. The *Shigella* organisms are excreted for 1–2 weeks, and intermittent excretion may be prolonged for more than a month in a proportion of cases—perhaps 20%, but it is difficult to distinguish examples of prolonged carriage from cases of re-infection in family and school groups.

## II. WATER-BORNE DISEASES

### Cholera

Cholera is an acute and severe disease caused by *Vibrio cholerae* or the related *Vibrio eltor*. These are Gram-negative curved bacteria. The source is a human case and spread is via water or food (Fig. 9.2). *V. cholerae* is non-invasive but produces an enterotoxin that causes a rapid outpouring of fluid and electrolytes from the gut mucosa. In treatment, fluid and electrolyte replacement is of

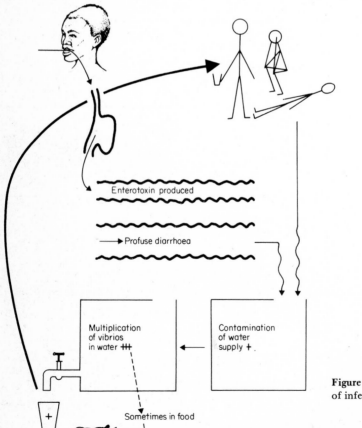

Enterotoxin produced

→ Profuse diarrhoea

Multiplication of vibrios in water +++

Contamination of water supply +

Sometimes in food

**Figure 9.2** The cycle of infection in cholera.

66

paramount importance and antibiotic therapy is of secondary importance. Cholera can be rapidly fatal and death is by dehydration from the vast loss of isotonic fluid in the stool (described as 'rice-water stool'). Prevention is by the provision of a safe water supply and a separate sewage disposal system. Vaccines containing killed cholera vibrios are available for active immunization, and an internationally recognized vaccination certificate is required by travellers in certain areas of the world. The degree of protection afforded by cholera vaccine to a traveller under such circumstances is short-lived and of debatable degree. Re-vaccination is required every 6 months. Better cholera vaccines are clearly needed, but the essential approach to prevention involves sewage engineering and the provision of safe drinking water.

**Typhoid Fever**

Typhoid fever (enteric fever) is caused by *Salmonella typhi*. The infection is usually acquired directly by drinking contaminated water (Fig. 9.3), though an outbreak in Aberdeen involved canned meat that had been contaminated by water used in a South American processing plant. The ultimate source of the

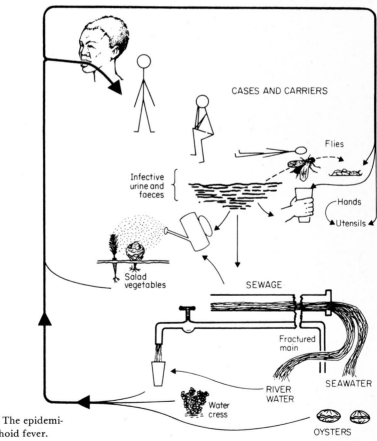

**Figure 9.3**  The epidemiology of typhoid fever.

disease is another human case or carrier of the infection. Unlike the other salmonellae, of which there are very many pathogenic sero-types, the typhoid bacillus does not naturally infect animals; typhoid fever is specifically a disease of man.

After ingestion under circumstances that afford some protection from the normal gastric acid barrier, the organism localizes in the lymphoid tissue of the small gut and multiplies. Invasion into the bloodstream occurs and there is a phase of bacteriaemia when the organism may be isolated from the blood. The liver is affected and the bacillus may set up a local infection in the gall-bladder. The organism is returned to the gut, via the bile, and there follows a phase of active proliferation in the lymphoid tissue with the development of longitudinal shallow ulcers. At this stage typhoid bacilli are abundant in the faeces. Renal involvement in the generalized infection may occur with the bacteria occurring sporadically in the urine. Blood culture may yield the organism in the early phase of the illness (weeks 1-2), and stool culture at any stage but especially in the middle or later stages (weeks 2-3). An agglutination test for specific antibodies to *S. typhi* (the Widal test) normally indicates a low or negative level of antibody in the early stage of the disease and a 'rising titre' in the later stages or thereafter, but there are difficulties in the interpretation of the Widal test that limit its value; for example, agglutinins may occur in low concentration in normal sera.

The severity of the illness varies. The classical patient is severely ill with a hectic fever, a skin rash, abdominal signs and symptoms and various complications. The disease may be fatal. Convalescent patients may continue to excrete the organism for some weeks. Chronic carriers occur and these people excrete the organism irregularly and indefinitely. Although *S. typhi* is sensitive to various antimicrobial agents *in vitro*, successful treatment of the infection is most reliably achieved with chloramphenicol. It is worrying that some chloramphenicol-resistant strains have been encountered recently. Ampicillin is sometimes used.


## VIRUSES ACQUIRED BY INGESTION

Two viruses that merit special mention in this section are the virus of infectious hepatitis A and poliovirus.

### Viral Hepatitis

There are two forms of this, A and B; hepatitis B is discussed on p.56. The virus of hepatitis A is acquired by ingestion and it is spread by the faecal-oral route or indirectly in contaminated food from human cases or convalescent carriers. The incubation period of hepatitis A is shorter than that of B, but it may be quite long (15−40 days); the faeces of a carrier may continue to be infective for more than a year. The illness varies in severity; it can present as an unpleasant subacute or acute fever with anorexia (loss of appetite) and nausea. The virus attacks the liver and jaundice develops. This disease is a recognized hazard for travellers in the Far East and it is known that a dose of human gamm-globulin affords useful passive protection for a few months.

## Poliomyelitis

There are three types of poliovirus (1, 2, 3) and these are immunologically distinct. They are enteroviruses acquired by ingestion and they localize in the lymphoid tissue of the oro-pharynx or gut; viral multiplication may then lead to a viraemia (virus in the blood). All of this may pass unnoticed, but in a small proportion of infections the virus causes damage in the central nervous system and this may lead to various paralyses. Transmission is from human to human by the faecal-oral route. In a non-immunized community, a vast reservoir of infection builds up; this largely consists of people who have been sub-clinically infected at some time in the past, and there will also be cases and convalescent carriers; the endemic infection is, in time, particularly likely to strike the young non-immune section or the non-immune visitor. Thus, poliomyelitis was called infantile paralysis in the past and the disease is presently recognized as a hazard to the non-immunized traveller in underdeveloped societies. Polio vaccines are noted on pp.108–111.

## A NOTE ON BACTERIAL CHALLENGES IN THE GUT

### Infections associated with a low challenge dose

A few organisms have specific infective potential at relatively low challenge doses and these may be carried on hands or passively in food or drink to produce new cases. Bacillary dysentery is a fairly convincing example of a hand-to-mouth infection, sometimes associated with mediate contact but not typically associated with food or drink. Other infective hazards at relatively low dose include typhoid fever and some cases of *Escherichia coli* gastroenteritis which is an acute and dangerous disease typically affecting infants and caused by so-called enteropathogenic strains of *Esch. coli.*

At the present stage of our ignorance, these diseases can be grouped together on the basis of their hand-to-mouth infectivity or their 'passive transfer' in food or drink, though a clinical bacteriologist, a clinician and an epidemiologist would all argue that these diseases are poles apart. The term 'passive transfer' is coined here to denote transfer without multiplication in the vehicle, but a multiplication stage in food can certainly occur and the challenge could then be even more severe.

Gastro-intestinal infections that can be transmitted by small challenge doses are characteristically difficult to control and are associated with a tendency to spread with the production of secondary cases, despite modern toilet systems. Our lack of care in this context is deplorable, and the design and use of the 'modern' toilet system in general take inadequate note of hygienic principles (see Fig. 9.1). This is also true of our catering.

### Infections associated with larger challenge doses

Infections that seem to be associated with moderately large challenge doses under certain circumstances include brucellosis, cholera, and *Vibrio parahaemolyticus* food poisoning (p.77), with milk, water and fish as the respective vehicles involved. It might be helpful to consider that these diseases, possibly involving quantitatively significant challenges, are 'actively transferred' in their vehicles. The diseases occur when circumstances allow a fairly large challenge to be delivered, but control can be achieved by relatively simple hygienic practices such as pasteurization, sewage engineering, and cold storage.

### Infections involving very large challenge doses

These are considered in the following chapter on bacterial food poisoning.

## A NOTE ABOUT WATER

An assured safe water supply is of paramount importance in the prevention of gastro-intestinal and other diseases. The filtration and chlorination of drinking water provide essential safeguards. In the routine bacteriological examination of water, attempts are not generally made to isolate and identify a specific pathogen. Rather, the bacteriologists enumerate coliform organisms in a test sample and assess the proportion that is really typical of *Esch. coli.* The latter are assumed to be of animal or human faecal origin and this gives a good indication of the degree of potentially dangerous contamination of the supply.

Water and wet things worry bacteriolgoists concerned with disease. Typhoid and cholera are classical examples of water-borne infection (p.66), but the association of water with potential trouble goes much further. Whereas dry materials are generally safe against microbial attack, wet or damp substances are liable to spoilage unless antimicrobial conditions are generated by salts, or sugars or other agents. Moreover, organisms can survive on wet surfaces in toilets or in kitchens or in wet areas of ward side-rooms to become serious dangers to new hosts. Dry skin is a fairly effective barrier against bacteria, but 'waterlogged' skin is vulnerable to fungal, bacterial, spirochaetal and viral attack. One of the major factors in the control of infection of burned patients is the susceptibility of an exuding surface to microbial colonization.

# 10 Bacterial food poisoning

Bacterial food poisoning is acute gastro-enteritis resulting from the ingestion of food or drink contaminated with certain bacteria or their toxic products (see Table 10.1).

**Table 10.1** Percentage occurrence of bacteria causing food poisoning in Britain in recent years (1969—1973).* (See Vernon, E. and Tillett, H.E., 1974.)

| | |
|---|---|
| Salmonellae (especially *S. typhimurium*) | *c.* 80 |
| *Clostridium welchii* | *c.* 15 |
| *Staphylococcus aureus* | *c.* 4 |
| *Escherichia coli* | 1-2 |
| *Bacillus cereus* | *c.* 0.5 |
| *Vibrio parahaemolyticus* | a few cases |
| *Streptococcus faecalis* | a few cases |
| *Clostridium botulinum* | 0 |

* Data from PHLS reports on *c.*40,000 cases in which a bacterial cause was identified: there are many food-poisoning incidents for which no recognized bacterial cause is identified.

Various infections such as typhoid fever and cholera and even dysentery can be transmitted via food or drink, but the term does not normally embrace these specific infections; they are listed in Table 10.2 and they are included in Table 10.3. Other bacteria that are involved when food 'goes off' or decomposes, the food-spoilage organisms, are not characteristically associated with disease and are not considered here.

As we change our habits of living, new mechanisms of microbial pathogenicity become apparent. It is quite likely that much of our food is contaminated with various organisms, but the challenge dose—the dose ingested by any one person—should be generally low. However, if bacteria are allowed to multiply in food, the challenge dose may become very high (Fig. 10.1). We now accept bulk cooking of foods and, in turn, bulk handling and processing of our foodstuffs. We readily accept communal eating, and we have been too ready to accept poor standards of food hygiene. Many canteens, catering establishments and domestic kitchens are now warm, and they contrast markedly with the cold sculleries of former years. If bacterial multiplication in food is to be avoided, provision of adequate chilling and refrigeration facilities is essential. Every household makes use of processed food, and every household should have a refrigerator in which to store products that are so vulnerable to bacterial contamination and growth. Some organisms such as *Clostridium botulinum* type E can grow and produce

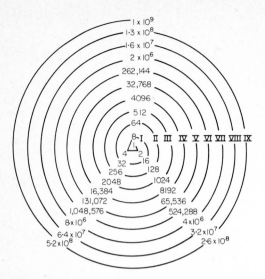

**Figure 10.1** A 'bacteriological clock' based on a generation time of 20 minutes. The Arabic numerals spiralling from the centre indicate the increase in numbers of organisms at 20-minute intervals. The Roman numerals indicate time in hours. [From Collee, 1974.]

lethal toxin at low temperatures and various psychrophilic food-spoilage organisms can grow in the refrigerator, but let us concentrate at present on the more common food poisoning patterns.

Bacterial growth and toxigenesis are related to time and temperature. It is important to bear in mind the following points: (i) Some raw foods such as milk, and many cooked or processed foods, can be a good culture medium when water is available in them for bacterial growth. (ii) Extremes of temperature kill at the upper limits but not at the bottom of the thermometer scale (Fig. 10.2). (iii) Bacterial spores often survive heating; 'heat-shock' may help them to germinate. (iv) Heat penetration into a bulk food and subsequent heat loss are slow processes, while the food passes through the 'incubation danger zone' in which bacteria may multiply readily.

Features of various food-borne diseases are listed in Table 10.3 and the following text is clearly an over-simplification. The term bacterial food poisoning tends to be restricted to circumstances in which the food or drink has provided a booster stage during which a contaminating dose of organisms may be transformed to an effective challenge in terms of infectivity or toxicity (Fig. 10.3). Thus, the recognized food-poisoning syndromes may be grouped as infective or toxic, though a third group exists in which there is an initial infective stage followed by the release of toxin in the gut.

## THE INFECTION TYPE

The classical cause of this type of food poisoning are members of the *Salmonella* genus, excluding the typhoid bacillus (*S. typhi*) which specifically causes

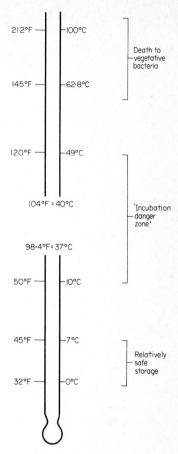

**Figure 10.2** Holding temperatures in relation to the hazard of growth of mesophilic bacteria in food. [From Collee, 1974.]

enteric fever in man (p.67) and does not naturally infect animals. However, a vast number of other salmonellae cause natural infections in a wide range of animals and birds and some of these organisms regularly cause food poisoning in man. Rodents are notorious carriers of salmonellae and *S. typhimurium*, the cause of 'mouse typhoid', is a virulent pathogen of man. *S. typhimurium* infects a wide range of other animal species and it is the *commonest single identified cause of bacterial food poisoning in Britain*. The ultimate source of trouble is characteristically an infected animal or bird or a human case or carrier of the infection. The chief animal reservoirs of salmonellae are cattle, fowls and pigs. It is difficult to think of a creature that is not a potential risk; the extensive list of animal sources embraces African lizards, cockroaches and a Persian crow.

The bulk processing of food and food ingredients coupled with bulk catering and our dependence on intensive rearing of livestock make us and our

73

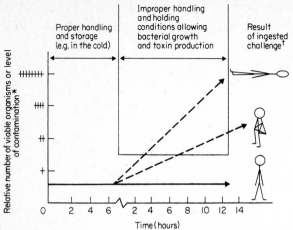

**Figure 10.3** The influence of time and temperature and the booster stage of bacterial contamination of food.

\* Bacterial multiplication is such that the level of contamination increases logarithmically (see Figure 10.1).

† See Table 10.3; in some cases, the production of disease depends upon the size of the challenge dose.

animals increasingly at risk from salmonella infection. Eggs and egg products may carry salmonellae and imported bulk egg must be pasteurized. Latent salmonella infections in cattle may flare up with the stress of calving or under the rigours of transport when calves typically fall sick. Contamination of pens at market and at abattoirs must be a common occurrence. As infections in cattle are common, milk pasteurization is an essential safeguard for man. Imported animal products for fertilizers or animal feeding stuffs are commonly contaminated with salmonellae and more control is needed here.

If food such as processed meat is contaminated with salmonellae and held under warm conditions, very large numbers of salmonellae are produced and the food becomes infective for man. On ingestion, sufficient numbers pass the gastric acid barrier. There is an incubation period of about a day while the

**Table 10.2** Specific diseases that may be transmitted via food, milk or water.

| |
|---|
| Typhoid and paratyphoid (the enteric fevers) |
| Brucellosis (undulant fever) |
| Bacillary dysentery (more usually associated with direct or mediate transfer) |
| Q fever (*Coxiella burnetii*) |
| Cholera |
| Tuberculosis (some forms) |
| Viral hepatitis A (infectious hepatitis) |
| Enteroviral diseases (often otherwise associated with air-borne transfer) — Polioviruses, Echoviruses, Coxsackie viruses |

organisms multiply further in the small intestine. Then symptoms and signs of an acute gastro-enteritis develop—nausea, vomiting, diarrhoea, stomach pains and fever.

The severity of the disease produced in man is variable. It may be virtually symptomless; it is frequently of considerable severity; it may be fulminating and it can be fatal. The organism occurs in the faeces of cases, but it also occurs in faeces of symptomless *carriers* who may have had a previously recognized illness or who may be unaware that they have acquired an intestinal pathogen.

Isolation and identification of salmonellae requires a complex series of bacteriological and serological procedures. Many hundreds of types of *Salmonella* are now recognizable and it is necessary to determine the exact identity of a type involved in an outbreak if the source of infection is to be

**Table 10.3**  A provisional guide to some features of the causative organisms of various food-borne diseases.

| Disease | Transmission | Infective challenge dose involved | Invasiveness | Known toxic challenge* |
|---|---|---|---|---|
| Bacillary dysentery | Hand-to-mouth | + | Local | — |
| Typhoid fever | 'Passive' in water, milk or food | + | General | —† |
| *Escherichia coli* gastro-enteritis | ? Passive in food, | ? +, ++ or +++ | Local or nil§ | — or + (*in vivo*) |
| Brucellosis | milk or | ++ | General | — |
| Cholera | water | ++ | — | + (*in vivo*) |
| *Vibro parahaemolyticus* food poisoning | 'Active' in food | ++ | — | + (*in vivo*) |
| *Salmonella* food poisoning | Booster stage in food or milk | +++ | Local‡ | —† |
| *Clostridium welchii* food poisoning | Booster stage in food | +++ | — | + (*in vivo*) |
| Staphylococcal food poisoning | Booster stage in food or milk | — | — | ++ (EXO) (N) |
| *Bacillus cereus* food poisoning | Booster stage in food | — | — | ++ (EXO) |
| Botulism | Booster stage in food | — | — | +++ (EXO) (N) |

* '*In vivo*' here indicates that toxin is elaborated within the gut; 'EXO' indicates that a known exotoxin is recognized; 'N' indicates neurotoxic activity.

† The endotoxins of various pathogenic Gram-negative bacteria are toxic, but the pathogenicity of these organisms is not solely attributable to their production of endotoxin.

‡ Some of the food-poisoning salmonellae, notably S. *typhimurium*, are occasionally invasive.

§ E. *coli* may be fiercely invasive in the neonate or young child.

— = nil or not recognized.

+, ++, +++ = increasing numbers of viable organisms (challenge dose) or increasing severity of toxic challenge.

traced. Although this at first appears to be a drawback, the variety of types that now exist allows the laboratory to be of real help to the epidemiologist and to the Public Health authorities in tracing any outbreak.

## TOXIC TYPES OF BACTERIAL FOOD POISONING

When *Staphylococcus aureus* grows in food, a powerful toxin may be produced; there are five serologically different staphylococcal enterotoxins A, B, C, D, E. On ingestion, the pre-formed toxin is absorbed and rapidly gives rise to acute symptoms that include vertigo, nausea, vomiting, diarrhoea and collapse. The interval between ingestion and onset of symptoms is typically short (1—6 hours).

Staphylococci are more salt-tolerant than most other pathogenic bacteria of man, and can therefore grow on salt cooked meat and cured meats. Processed or made-up meats are commonly involved in staphylococcal food poisoning. Other foods incriminated include custards, trifles and milk products.

Staphylococci may gain access to food from the infected hand of a food-handler, or from a hand that has been contaminated with staphylococci present in the nose of the food-handler. The organisms may also be derived from animal sources such as the cow, but pasteurization of milk reduces this hazard. Human sources of staphylococci are therefore most likely to be involved.

Staphylococcal food poisoning is an acute and very unpleasant illness; it is responsible for about 1—4 per cent of all cases. Caterers must learn to accept that this potentially dangerous organism is regularly carried by man and they must ensure that food is not held under conditions that allow staphylococci to multiply and produce toxin.

It is clearly unacceptable to allow people with staphylococcal infections, such as boils and whitlows, to come into contact with food. Waterproof adhesive plasters may resist wetting, but ventilated types are likely to shed large numbers of organisms. As ventilated dressings are advisable for efficient healing, the only way around the impasse is to be off work until the wound has healed. This raises many economic problems.

*Botulism* affects man and animals. It is an intoxication, i.e. it follows ingestion of pre-formed toxin in food or drink, and it is often fatal. The causative organism is an anaerobic sporing bacillus, *Clostridium botulinum*. There are at least 6 different types (A—F) and each type produces an immunologically distinct toxin; antitoxin prepared against type-A will not protect against type-B, for example. By such toxin-neutralization tests, the organisms or the pre-formed toxin may be typed. The types associated with botulism in man are types A and B, which occur widely in soil, and type E which is associated with fish and marine products. The spores are resistant to deleterious influences such as heat or drying. When the organism multiplies in food under suitable conditions it may produce botulinum toxin. This potent neurotoxin causes various paralyses and upsets of the nervous system and there is a typical clinical picture.

*Bacillus cereus* is a widely distributed aerobic spore-forming bacillus associated with a form of Chinese Restaurant food poisoning. The organism grows

76

in left-over cooked rice and produces a toxin that gives rise to an acute food-poisoning syndrome when it is eaten.

*Vibrio parahaemolyticus*, a halophilic (salt-loving) organism that multiplies in warm sea-water, can cause food poisoning by producing toxin in uncooked fish which is eaten raw.

## A TOXI-INFECTIVE TYPE OF BACTERIAL FOOD POISONING

*Clostridium welchii* is a large bacillus that will grow only in the absence of oxygen. It dies on exposure to air, but it can produce spores that will survive. These spores are widely distributed in dirt, faeces, flies, meat, etc. Some of them are particularly resistant to heat. When such spores are present in meat during cooking they frequently survive. The meat ensures an anaerobic medium and during the cooling stage the organisms germinate and multiply to produce enormous numbers in a few hours ($10^7$-$10^8$ per ml).

*Survival* of spores is ensured by initially heavy contamination and by inadequate heat penetration. *Germination* is activated by heat shock and is encouraged by the anaerobic environment of cooked meat. *Growth* is enhanced by an abundance of soluble nutrients in a progressively anaerobic environment. A prolonged cooling period within a suitable temperature range allows rapid and continued bacterial multiplication. Victims therefore ingest a cooked meat broth culture containing millions of viable *Cl. welchii*. It appears that the organisms sporulate in the gut and release an enterotoxin at this stage. Symptoms of abdominal pain and diarrhoea occur 8—24 hours after ingestion of the meal.

Typical features of an outbreak of *Cl. welchii* food poisoning are thus:
(1)   Pre-cooked or bulk-cooked meat is usually involved.
(2)   There is an incubation period of about 12 hours.
(3)   Symptoms include abdominal pains and diarrhoea. Fever and vomiting are not typically produced.
(4)   Symptoms usually subside after 24—48 hours.
(5)   The causative organism can be isolated from the food concerned and from the faeces of the victims.
Meals served in schools, hospitals and canteens tend to be mainly involved in the *Cl. welchii* outbreaks. The occurrence of *Cl. welchii* food poisoning is a serious reflection on the unhygienic practices of the catering establishments concerned.

### The challenge of diagnosis

It has been necessary to limit this discussion to certain bacterial diseases, and to exclude other conditions such as abdominal tuberculosis, streptococcal disease and Q fever that can be food-borne. Moreover, the medical practitioner must also be aware of viral, protozoal, fungal, algal and chemical causes of disease that may present with gastro-intestinal signs and symptoms. The differential diagnosis is complex. Clinical appearances suggestive of a cerebro-vascular attack or of coronary thrombosis may be produced by staphylococcal food-poisoning or botulism; and the syndrome of staphylococcal food poisoning can be produced by a viral infection known as winter vomiting disease. Prompt diagnosis can be of vital importance, and an efficient epidemiological service ensuring communication between practitioners, clinicians, public health officers and laboratory workers is essential.

Further research is also needed. In recent investigations of gastro-enteritis in young children, the virologists have discovered a bewildering series of particles variously named *rheovirus*-like, *orbiviruses, rotaviruses, duoviruses* and *astroviruses*. Whilst *Escherichia coli* is an acknowledged bacterial pathogen in this field, it is likely that certain enteropathogenic viruses will be more clearly defined in the near future. This could help to account for at least some of the many cases of diarrhoeal disease that have many of the features of an infection but which presently lack a label.

# 11 Zoonoses

Diseases transmitted from animals to man are grouped under this heading (Table 11.1). The following list is not intended to be exhaustive but to illustrate biological versatility and some occupational hazards in relation to host-parasite associations.

## FUNGAL DISEASES TRANSMITTED FROM ANIMALS TO MAN

Various mycotic infections of animals may affect man. Common examples are some ringworm conditions caused by dermatophytic fungi that are pathogenic for man and animals. Such fungi with an affinity for animals are referred to as zoophilic. They tend to be transmitted to man, often to children, by direct or mediate contact. For example, cattle rubbing themselves on posts may transfer fungi from their skin lesions to surfaces that are subsequently likely to implant an infective dose into the skin of a farm-worker or a visitor.

## BACTERIAL DISEASES TRANSMITTED FROM ANIMALS TO MAN

### Anthrax
This is the classical example. It is a serious septicaemic illness of herbivorous animals. The anthrax bacillus is an aerobic Gram-positive sporing rod and the resistance of its spores ensures that potentially dangerous numbers of organisms can survive in an infected pasture, on an infected animal skin or hide, or in infected animal bones or bone meal. Control of the first hazard is achieved in this country by special rules governing the notification of anthrax in animals and the disposal of the carcase. Trouble associated with the second hazard is minimized by strict control of the importation of animal hides and skins into Britain, by restriction of their importation to one port (Liverpool), and by the provision of facilities there for their disinfection. The third hazard is recognized, and some practices such as the autoclaving of bone meal take account of it—but this control is not yet rigid and some farmers and amateur gardeners have contracted anthrax as a result of handling bone meal.

When anthrax spores are implanted on an abrasion of the skin, they produce a local lesion called a 'malignant pustule' with a black crust; anthrax is Greek for coal. Unless this is treated promptly, the organisms thereafter become highly invasive and produce a fatal septicaemic illness. This form of the disease was significantly referred to as 'Hide Porter's disease'. In the bad old days before the Factory Acts, pulmonary anthrax acquired by inhalation of air-borne spores was called 'Woolsorter's disease'.

**Table 11.1**   Various zoonoses caused by fungi, bacteria, spirochaetes, rickettsiae and viruses.

| PATHOGENIC ORGANISM | ANIMAL SOURCE | INFECTION IN MAN |
|---|---|---|
| Dermatophytic fungi | Domesticated animals and pets | Ringworm (tinea) |
| *Cryptococcus neoformans* | Pigeons | Cryptococcal meningitis (torulosis) |
| *Bacillus anthracis* | Herbivorous animals | Anthrax |
| *Brucella* spp. (*abortus, melitensis, suis*) | Sheep, cattle, goats, pigs | Brucellosis (Undulant Fever) |
| *Salmonella* spp. (*typhimurium, enteritidis, dublin* etc.) | Cattle, poultry, pigs, rodents and many others | Salmonellosis (food poisoning) and other syndromes |
| *Mycobacterium bovis* and *M. avium* | Cattle, pigs | Tuberculosis (some forms) |
| *Yersinia pestis* | Rats and other rodents | Plague |
| *Leptospira* spp. | Rodents, dogs, pigs | Leptospirosis (Weil's disease and other forms, e.g. canicola fever) |
| *Rickettsia* spp. | Arthropods | Typhus and related fevers |
| *Coxiella burnetii* | Cattle, sheep, goats | Q fever |
| Chlamydia organisms | Birds | Ornithosis; psittacosis |
| *Vaccinia virus* | Cattle | Cowpox |
| Virus B (herpesvirus simiae) | Monkeys | Acute paralytic illness |
| LC-virus (an arenavirus) | Mice | Lymphocytic chorio-meningitis |
| Arboviruses | Various vertebrates — associated with various arthropods | Yellow Fever and other diseases |
| Rabies virus | Various carnivores and bats | Rabies |

## Brucellosis

Brucella organisms are small Gram-negative cocco-bacilli that cause disease in sheep, cattle, goats and pigs. Man generally becomes infected by ingestion of milk from infected cows or goats, by handling infected meat, or by handling infected animals. The disease produced in man is undulant fever—a recurrent pyrexial illness with a range of clinical features. It is typically associated with the unwise drinking of unpasteurized milk, particularly goat's milk in the Mediterranean littoral, but it is also an occupational hazard of butchers, farmers and veterinary surgeons—especially in relation to direct contact with the products of conception when cows are calving; these tissues are rich in erythritol which promotes the growth of the brucella organisms and accounts for their enrichment in the animal, but not the human, placenta.

## Salmonellosis
We have said quite enough of salmonella infections and their animal sources at p.73 to make the point that these are most important infections transmitted from animals to man. Note that *Salmonella typhi* does not have an animal host other than man (p.67).

## Tuberculosis
Mycobacteria closely related to *Mycobacterium tuberculosis* cause tuberculous disease in cattle and pigs. These organisms can also cause disease in man. The usual mode of infection is by ingestion of infected unpasteurized cows' milk and the form of tuberculosis that then arises in man is abdominal, affecting the gut and mesenteric lymph nodes—sometimes also involving pelvic organs and sometimes affecting bones and joints. The disease has been controlled in Britain by tuberculin-testing of herds and removal of infected animals and by pasteurization of milk. Bovine strains of tubercle bacilli can also cause pulmonary disease in man if the organisms are inhaled.

## Plague
A small Gram-negative cocco-bacillus with characteristic polar staining is the cause of plague—a disease of rats and man. The organism used to be called *Pasteurella pestis* but is now classified as *Yersinia pestis*. The primary natural hosts are rats and other rodents. Endemic infection in the wild rodent population is transmitted by their associated fleas and becomes more intensive and widespread if the flea population increases. Fleas of the *Xenopsylla* species are typically involved and their numbers have seasonal increases when local climatic conditions are favourable for them. The disease then extends from the wild rodents to rats associated with human habitations, notably the black rat, *Rattus Rattus*. When these hosts succumb, some of the fleas bearing an infected blood meal may transfer to nearby human hosts. The plague bacilli meanwhile multiply and block the proventriculus of the flea and the organisms are injected into the new host at its next attempt to feed.

Initially, the infection is localized at a regional lymph gland and the swollen node is referred to as a bubo, hence 'bubonic plague'. There may be subsequent invasion with dark haemorrhagic effusions—'the Black Death'. If the respiratory involvement is clinically evident or if the lungs are involved and there is transmission to another victim by the respiratory route, the condition is referred to as 'pneumonic plague'. The distinction between bubonic and pneumonic plague is made much of in textbooks, but people with practical experience of plague stress that the disease may produce a spectrum of different syndromes of varying severity.

## Leptospirosis

Spirochaetes of the genus *Leptospira* are widely distributed in nature. They are all grouped in a complex referred to as *L. interrogans* of which saprophytic (non-pathogenic) serotypes form the *biflexa* sub-group. The pathogenic serotypes, which include those formerly recognized as *L. canicola* and *L. icterohaemorrhagiae*, have animal hosts and may cause diseases in man that range from a relatively mild feverish illness with features of meningitis (canicola fever) to a dangerously severe illness with hectic fever, jaundice and haemorrhagic features (Weil's disease). A mild canicola-like illness with vague malaise may occur in piggery-workers or in those who handle dogs; the pig and the dog can act as the natural host. However, small rodents are more widely and more frequently involved as the natural hosts of other pathogenic leptospirae and they form an important world-wide reservoir of infection. For example, the *icterohaemorrhagiae* serotype is carried by the brown rat; when rats are infected with such leptospirae, they excrete the organisms in their urine and the infection may then be transmitted to man. Occupational hazards of this sort threaten such groups as miners working in wet pits in which rats are abundant or sugar-cane workers in wet fields that harbour rodents.

## RICKETTSIAL DISEASES AND COXIELLA INFECTION TRANSMITTED TO MAN

The rickettsiae are essentially intracellular parasites that are harboured by various arthropods, including lice, ticks and mites. The bite of an infected arthropod may transmit the disease to man, or the agent may be 'scratched-in' from arthropod faeces when man scratches the area on his skin. Examples of the rickettsiae involved and their arthropod vectors are given in Table 11.2.

The diagnosis of rickettsial disease rests upon the laboratory isolation of

**Table 11.2**   Some examples of pathogenic rickettsiae and their arthropod vectors.

| Infective agent | Arthropod vector | Disease in man |
|---|---|---|
| *R. prowazekii* | Body louse | Epidemic typhus |
| *R. mooseri* | Rat flea | Endemic typhus |
| *R. rickettsii* | Tick | Rocky Mountain spotted fever |
| *R. australis* | Tick | Queensland typhus |
| *R. tsutsugamushi* | Mite | Scrub typhus |

the organism (a potentially hazardous exercise) and on the serological demonstration of complement-fixing antibodies in the patient's blood. It so happens that, as some rickettsiae have haptens in common with certain variants of *Proteus vulgaris* and *P. mirabilis*, the serum of a patient with a rickettsial disease may contain agglutinins for these *Proteus* organisms. This is the basis of the *Weil-Felix* reaction.

Q fever is caused by a rickettsia-like agent called *Coxiella burnetii*. This feverish illness is usually transmitted by inhalation of infected droplets or dust contaminated with the excretions or secretions of infected cattle, sheep or goats, or by ingestion of infected raw milk. The agent is slightly heat-resistant but normal pasteurization procedures are likely to reduce the challenge dose to a non-infective level.

## Ornithosis

This is a general term for a group of diseases acquired from birds and caused by chlamydia organisms (p.1). The classical example is *psittacosis* which occurs in parrots and budgerigars; related diseases occur in pigeons, poultry and some sea-birds. Psittacosis in man may arise when infected dust or droplets are inhaled. There may be a flu-like illness and a form of pneumonia may develop.

## VIRAL DISEASES TRANSMITTED FROM ANIMALS TO MAN

A classical example is *cowpox*. The antigenic relationship of the causative virus to smallpox virus was turned greatly to man's advantage by Jenner's development of vaccination. Smallpox does not generally occur in animals and that disease spreads primarily from man to man, but cowpox virus can spread by contact from the cow to the hand of the dairyman or farm-worker. Jenner noted that those who had suffered from cowpox were subsequently resistant to smallpox. The virus now used for the prevention of smallpox is derived from cowpox virus.

## Virus B

A herpes virus affecting monkeys (herpes virus simiae) may be transmitted by bite or by other routes to laboratory workers. A very severe and potentially fatal neurological disease ensues in man under these circumstances.

## Lymphocytic choriomeningitis

The virus of *lymphocytic choriomeningitis*, an arenavirus (a particle resembling a grain of sand), occurs in mice and may be transmitted to man by inhalation of dust that has been contaminated with mouse excretions or secretions. The disease in man may present as a meningitis or as a feverish illness with respiratory signs and symptoms.

### The Arboviruses

Several important virus groups are linked under this heading because they are *arthropod-borne.* The viruses multiply in the tissues of the arthropod and are then transmitted when the arthropod bites its vertebrate host. These include the viruses of yellow fever, various encephalitis viruses, and some viruses associated with fevers that vary widely in their unpleasantness. This ecological grouping of quite different taxonomic groups of viruses can be misleading. The present comments are here limited to an example in which man is an important alternative vertebrate host to a mosquito that carries a dangerous virus: The example is *Yellow Fever.*

### Yellow Fever

The virus of yellow fever is carried from man to man by a mosquito *Aedes aegypti*; the disease varies in its severity, but the severe form is associated with jaundice resulting from liver damage and this may be rapidly fatal. A focus of infection occurs in the monkey population and is here transmitted by other mosquitoes which, on occasion, encounter man and pass the disease from the forest (sylvatic) phase to the domestic (urban) phase.

Immunization against yellow fever with an attenuated live virus preparation is effective and durable for at least 10 years.

### Rabies

This disease can be transmitted to man by the bite of an affected dog or wolf; cats and other feline species are another source, and various other animals including foxes can be involved. The virus is also harboured by vampire bats in South America and may affect cattle bitten by them.

The virus travels from the site of entry to affect the central nervous system and the disease in man is associated with delirious uncontrolled movements and an inability to swallow water without choking (hence 'hydrophobia', a colourful name for the disease). Eosinophilic inclusion bodies (Negri bodies) are produced in affected nerve cells and these are best seen in the hippocampus area of the brain. The established disease is almost invariably fatal.

Prevention of the disease depends upon rigid enforcement of quarantine measures and eradication of affected animals. If a person is licked or bitten by an animal thought to have rabies, it is important to secure the animal for observation and to protect the person by a series of active and passive immunizing procedures.

# 12 Sterilization, disinfection and asepsis

*Sterility* denotes the complete absence of micro-organisms—protozoa, fungi, bacteria and viruses. It is only achieved in normal clinical practice by special attention to detail in the processing of certain items. In many instances the word is wrongly applied; truly *sterile* instruments or articles have usually been subjected to dry heat at 160°C for 1 hour, or to wet heat in the autoclave at 121°C for 15-20 minutes, or to carefully monitored gamma radiation, or to a special gassing procedure with ethylene oxide, or to specified concentrations of formaldehyde or glutaraldehyde under controlled conditions. Many other procedures regularly used in clinical practice may *disinfect*, but few others are likely to guarantee sterility.

*Disinfection* denotes a marked reduction in the numbers of organisms present on an article, and this particularly relates to the exclusion of those that are likely to cause infection. Antiseptics are chemical disinfectants that may be allowed to come into contact with living tissues without unduly harming them. Such mild disinfectants cannot be expected to be promptly and effectively lethal to all forms of micro-organisms including bacterial spores (which are markedly resistant to chemical attack) and viruses (which are relatively resistant to some chemicals).

### Skin preparation for surgery

It is certainly not possible to sterilize living skin by the transient application of an antiseptic agent; for example, even many strong disinfectants do not inactivate certain pathogenic bacterial spores that can occur on skin. The best that a surgeon can normally hope to do before making an incision is to reduce the transient and resident flora at the operation site on the skin by thorough cleansing, and then to inactivate the accessible vegetative bacteria by applying 70 per cent ethanol (or better 70 per cent isopropyl alcohol) in water. Another antiseptic may be incorporated with the spirit, such as chlorhexidine or iodine, but it is the alcohol that achieves a quick kill. It is important that the alcohol is 70 per cent *in water*.

## A SUMMARY OF COMMON MEDICAL APPLICATIONS OF CHEMICAL ANTISEPTICS AND DISINFECTANTS

The following list is incomplete, but it helps to illustrate currently observed practices and principles.

(1) *For skin cleansing*
    (i) Soap and water, *or*
    (ii) Detergent preparations such as Teepol or laurolinium, *or*
    (iii) Quaternary ammonium compounds such as cetrimide or benzalkonium chloride (Fig. 12.1).

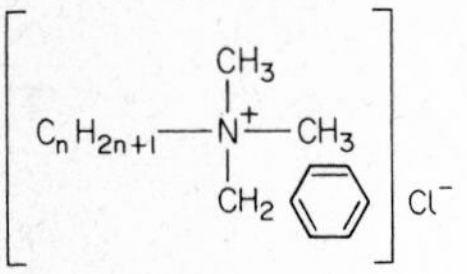

**Figure 12.1**    BENZALKONIUM CHLORIDE—
a quaternary ammonium compound (n = 8 − 18).

(2) *For a slowly cumulative antibacterial effect on skin*
    Hexachlorophane (with appropriate precautions) (Fig. 12.2).

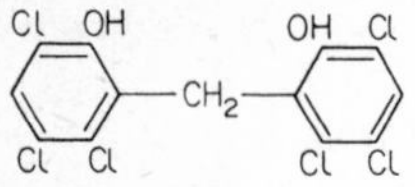

**Figure 12.2**    HEXACHLOROPHANE.

(3) *For rapid pre-operative disinfection of skin*
    70% isopropyl alcohol (or 70% ethanol) with 30% water + chlorhexidine 1% (Fig. 12.3) or iodine 2%.

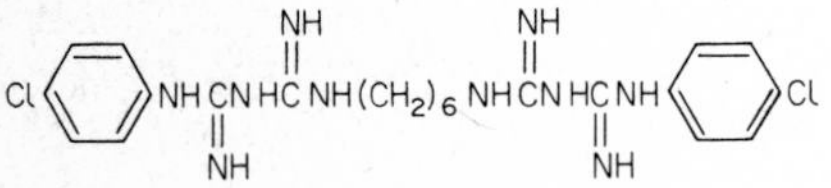

**Figure 12.3**    CHLORHEXIDINE.

(4) *For more prolonged (planned) pre-operative disinfection of the skin*
    Povidone-iodine compresses.

(5) *For local application to contaminated tissues*
    (i) Chloroxylenol cream (Dettol),
    (ii) Chlorhexidine cream (Hibitane),
    (iii) Cetrimide cream (Savlon),
    (iv) Acridine or rosaniline dyes (e.g. flavine).

(6) *For local application to infected tissues*
    (i) Chlorhexidine,
    (ii) Silver nitrate (for selected burns cases),
    (iii) Hypochlorite solution,

(iv) neomycin-bacitracin (with precautions as these are antibiotics).

(7) *For disinfecting clean drinking water*
Chlorine.

(8) *For disinfecting clean (inanimate) surfaces*
   (i) Hypochlorite with detergent, *or*
   (ii) 70% ethanol with 30% water, *or*
   (iii) 70% isopropyl alcohol with 30% water.

(9) *For disinfecting dirty surfaces*
Floors, toilets, etc. ('coarse disinfection'):
Cresols—Sudol, Lysol.

*Note*
Phenol (carbolic acid) (Fig. 12.4) is toxic and its antimicrobial activity is greatly reduced when it is diluted. It is not used as a general disinfectant.

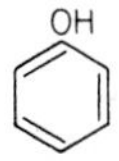

**Figure 12.4** PHENOL.

Phenolic disinfectants include cresol-containing coal-tar derivatives (Fig. 12.5) such as black fluid and Jeyes' fluid. They are effective for coarse disinfection of contaminated surfaces and lavatories. They retain their activity in the presence of organic matter, but their potential toxicity for man should be borne in mind.

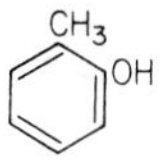

**Figure 12.5** ortho-CRESOL.

Chloroxylenol antiseptics (Fig. 12.6) such as Dettol are popular. They are inactivated by organic matter and are not suitable for coarse disinfection. They are often abused in this context—an expensive and ineffective exercise.

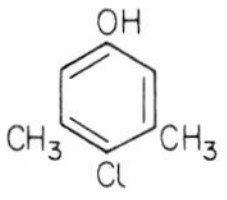

**Figure 12.6** CHLOROXYLENOL.

(10) *For sterilizing clean instruments or apparatus, equipment, etc.*
  (i)  Buffered glutaraldehyde fluid (Fig. 12.7), e.g. Cidex.
  (ii) Ethylene oxide gas (Fig. 12.8).

$CHO \cdot CH_2 \cdot CH_2 \cdot CH_2 \cdot CHO$

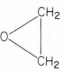

**Figure 12.7**  GLUTARALDEHYDE.

**Figure 12.8**  ETHYLENE OXIDE.

## ASEPSIS

Just as prevention is better than cure, so asepsis is better than antisepsis—and this demands the use of sterile instruments, dressings and suture materials. The surgeon's hands are also cleansed as thoroughly as possible, and then gloved because skin bacteria cannot otherwise be excluded. A cap, mask, theatre gown, light trousers and boots help to keep the surgeon's flora away from the patient, provided that the mask has an impermeable layer and the trousers are tucked into the boots. Various applications and sterile drapes are used in attempts to keep the patient's flora away from the operation site.

The surgical team is in turn masked and gowned and due attention is paid to the possibility of air-borne transmission of organisms into the operation wound. Plenum ventilation helps to avoid air-borne contamination (see Figs. 12.9, 12.10). Laminar air-flow systems may be used. Commercially designed surgical suites are now available as pre-fabricated units. Above all, the surgical

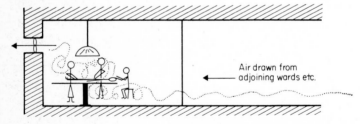

Air drawn from adjoining wards etc.

**Figure 12.9**  How *not* to ventilate a surgical theatre. An extractor system high in the theatre draws contaminated air up from the floor and in from adjoining treatment areas.

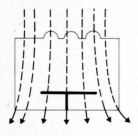

**Figure 12.10**  The aim of the plenum principle is to introduce clean air from above and to remove it at floor level while maintaining a slightly positive pressure within the theatre. Laminar flow devices operating over limited critical areas are now being developed.

instruments and equipment must be sterile (see below). Many hospitals have a Central Sterile Supply Unit with responsibility for the issuing of sterile pre-packed sets of surgical instruments and for the supply of smaller sterile packs that might range from a sterile syringe to an emergency tracheostomy set. The Unit also arranges for the collecting and sorting of contaminated items, with proper safeguards, and for the cleansing and re-sterilization of the non-disposable items.

## DISINFECTION AND STERILIZATION BY PHYSICAL METHODS

*Filtration.* Liquid preparations that would be damaged by heat, e.g. serum, antibiotic solutions, are often 'sterilized' by filtration. The filters, e.g. *Seitz filters* which employ replaceable asbestos disks, have pores so small that ordinary bacteria are arrested. Note that *viruses pass through*; for many laboratory purposes they can be ignored, but fluids rendered bacteria-free by Seitz or similar filtration must not be used for clinical injections.

*Pasteurization* kills vegetative cells of bacteria. It usually involves exposure to wet heat at temperatures of about 60-80°C for times ranging from 30 minutes to 30 seconds. The process must be most carefully monitored. Bacterial spores are *not* killed.

*Boiling.* If a clean instrument is held in boiling water for 5-10 minutes, it is normally freed of most significant pathogens. Its sterility is not guaranteed, however, and its early recontamination frequently results when it is handled wet and skin bacteria are carried into the film of water on its surface—often draining to the cutting edge or point of the instrument.

*The Autoclave* and the pressure cooker work on the same principle—that the temperature of pure steam under pressure rises above 100°C as the pressure is increased; at 1.05 kg/cm² (15 lbs per in²) it is 121°C. As wet heat is much more damaging to micro-organisms than dry heat, the autoclave combines this effect with the added advantage that any steam reaching a cool surface condenses and gives up latent heat at that point. Moreover, more steam is drawn in to take its place. Clearly any surface to be sterilized must be accessible to the steam; anyone attempting to autoclave articles in closed metal boxes, or impermeable powders and oils and ointments, betrays an ignorance of this elementary principle. It is essential that items for sterilization in an autoclave should be exposed to pure steam and that mixtures of air and steam are avoided.

At the end of a sterilization period of 15-20 minutes, a vacuum is sometimes pulled in a modern autoclave so that the load of dressings is dried. Some autoclaves work at higher pressures and thus achieve higher temperatures (still under conditions of wet heat); exposure times can be accordingly shorter, and it is wise to start with an evacuation step to remove most of the air and allow prompt access of steam. These autoclaves are referred to as 'pre-vacuum high-temperature (135°C) short-time instruments'.

*The Hot Air Oven.* Some articles, such as glassware or impermeable powders or greases, are more conveniently sterilized in the dry state by treatment in an oven, at 160°C for 1 hour. This is obviously unsuitable for goods such

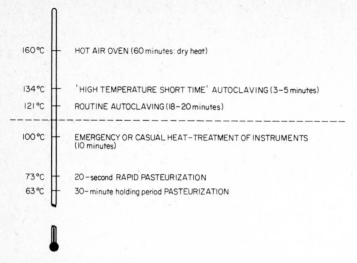

| | |
|---|---|
| 160°C | HOT AIR OVEN (60 minutes: dry heat) |
| 134°C | 'HIGH TEMPERATURE SHORT TIME' AUTOCLAVING (3–5 minutes) |
| 121°C | ROUTINE AUTOCLAVING (18–20 minutes) |
| 100°C | EMERGENCY OR CASUAL HEAT–TREATMENT OF INSTRUMENTS (10 minutes) |
| 73°C | 20–second RAPID PASTEURIZATION |
| 63°C | 30–minute holding period PASTEURIZATION |

**Figure 12.11** A summary of heat-treatment temperatures.

as rubber or plastic gloves and dressings that would char under these conditions.

*Ultra-violet Irradiation (UV).* Light at wavelengths of 240–330 nm is lethal to micro-organisms and viruses. It causes damage to the DNA that can be partly repaired on re-exposure to visible light by a process known as photo-reactivation. UV has very little penetrating power and organisms can be shielded by the equivalent of a thin sheet of paper. The application of UV as a disinfecting agent is therefore severely limited, but it may be used to reduce the bacterial and viral content of air and it is sometimes used to treat fluids by irradiation of thin films.

*Ionizing Radiations.* X-rays and gamma rays inactivate micro-organisms. A radioactive cobalt source ($^{60}$Co) can be used commercially to sterilize prepacked articles such as scalpel blades, plastic gloves and plastic syringes. The process is fairly slow and the necessary installation and shielding arrangements are costly. Ionizing radiation reduces the tensile strength of fibres.

# 13 Antimicrobial drugs: antibiotics and chemotherapeutic agents

The local or 'topical' application of antiseptic chemicals has been referred to in an earlier volume in this series (Vol. 1, p.101) and the concept of *selective toxicity* is noted particularly in relation to the more critical use of antimicrobial drugs to combat infections within the circulating fluids and tissues of the body. Here, the drug must have a special affinity for the micro-organism and must be relatively non-toxic to the cells of the human host. Substances used *in vivo* in this way are generally referred to as antibiotics or chemotherapeutic agents. The term 'antibiotic' is often used loosely to cover the whole range.

## PRINCIPLES OF USE

Antibiotics and chemotherapeutic agents are valuable and should be used with care. We must consider this in relation to the interests of the individual patient in whom an infective process may call for positive control or masterly inactivity on the part of the clinician who should attempt to recognize self-limiting infections. We must also consider our collective interest as a society in which the control of antibiotic resistance is of increasing importance. Each of us, at some time in our lives, is likely to require effective antimicrobial therapy; at that time, it will not be reassuring to learn that the value of the chosen agent has been much reduced by carelessness.

The properties of a hypothetical wonder drug 'Miraclomycin I' are outlined in Table 13.1. It is shown as one of a series, because each wonder drug would ideally have rather narrow specificity for a limited number of related pathogens. The properties listed in Table 13.1 indicate factors that we have come to value in various antimicrobial agents, but unfortunately few preparations have a good

Table 13.1    The properties of a hypothetical wonder drug.

Potently bactericidal
Cheap
Non-toxic, non-irritant, non-staining
Specific (narrow-spectrum)
High concentrations of active form obtainable in tissues
    —especially in blood, urine, CSF, bile, bone, brain
    and eye
No resistance or cross-resistance
No sensitization
No significant protein-binding
Effective orally, but absorbed proximally
Stable, but metabolized by man

proportion of these virtues.

Almost all of the significant work in the development of the clinically useful antibiotics has been done by pharmaceutical firms, and we can well understand why the industry must regard us at times as rather poor academic cousins with expensive ideals. There is, of course, an inevitable conflict between cautious control and a marketing policy that brings down prices and pays for further developments.

There are many valid reasons for not prescribing a drug to combat an infection and the decision to use an antibiotic should be supported by clearly positive reasons. Most cases of colds, flu and feverish chills, diarrhoea and food poisoning do not merit antibiotic therapy; in some cases the giving of an antibiotic can be shown to be clearly against the patient's interests.

## THE CHOICE

The microbiological report may be of great help to the clinician in selecting the right treatment, but the initial decision is often required promptly, before the laboratory report is available. In many circumstances, the clinician can base his first choice on a knowledge of the likely pathogens and their probable sensitivities. Local laboratory information based on recent experience can be of great help. For example, the data given in Table 13.2 show how the 'best-guess principle' might be applied in the initial treatment of a case of urinary tract infection occurring within the area surveyed.

Table 13.2 An antibiotic-sensitivity league table based on results with 6,080 strains (all species) of bacteria from out-patients and 17,411 strains from in-patients with urinary tract infections.

| Antibiotic* | Percentage no. of strains sensitive | |
| --- | --- | --- |
| | from out-patients | from in-patients |
| Cotrimoxazole | 93 | 88 |
| Nitrofurantoin | 88 | 82 |
| Nalidixic acid | 87 | 81 |
| Ampicillin | 79 | 63 |
| Sulphonamide | 65 | 56 |
| Tetracycline | 65 | 50 |

* The term antibiotic now tends to be applied loosely to all antimicrobial chemo-therapeutic agents.
From McAllister *et al.*, (1971); for full reference see Table 7.1.

Some organisms associated with certain illnesses are invariably or almost invariably sensitive to certain antibiotics. For example, the haemolytic streptococcus that causes follicular tonsillitis (streptococcal sore throat) is always sensitive to penicillin. On the other hand, the staphylococci that cause boils, carbuncles and wound infections, are often resistant to penicillin and it is necessary to have antibiotic sensitivity tests to guide the clinician. When an antibiotic has been properly selected, it is then important to ensure that an adequate dose is given by the proper route at the correct intervals over a sufficiently long period of time. The considerations that the clinician must have in mind before he decides on this action are outlined in Fig. 13.1, and the nature of the microbiological advice is also indicated.

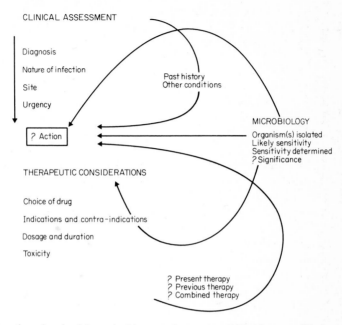

**Figure 13.1** Considerations involved in a decision to give or to withhold an antibiotic.

The factors that require consideration in an individual case are numerous and complex. In general, a bactericidal drug is preferable to one that is bacteriostatic and in some urgent cases this distinction may be critical.

Some antibiotics are effectively bactericidal; penicillin and streptomycin are good examples. Other antibiotics are almost purely bacteriostatic; this is true of chloramphenicol and essentially true for the tetracyclines. With some clear exceptions, it is often sufficient to produce a bacteriostatic effect which holds an infection in check and allows the host defences to regain control.

In many circumstances, the in-vitro evidence of sensitivity is endorsed by the clinical response to a particular antibiotic, but typhoid fever provides a good example of a situation in which the causative organism's sensitivity to various antibiotics in test-tube tests is not paralleled by clinical experience of patients' responses to the various antibiotics.

## ANTIBIOTIC SENSITIVITY TESTS

As a routine, the relative sensitivity of a bacterial strain to a particular antibiotic

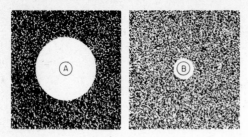

**Figure 13.2** Antibiotic disk sensitivity tests. A zone of inhibition of growth around disk A indicates a degree of sensitivity of the test organism to antibiotic A. A pattern of resistance is shown in relation to disk B.

is assessed by a *disk sensitivity test* (Fig. 13.2) in which a paper disk impregnated with the antibiotic at a known concentration is placed on an agar culture medium seeded with the test organism. The size of the zone of growth inhibition around the disk gives an index of sensitivity if various conditions are standardized. The test is performed in parallel with a standard bacterial strain of known sensitivity to provide a check. There are various modifications of this approach.

A more critical assessment of antibiotic sensitivity is obtained with a *tube-dilution procedure* (Fig. 13.3) which indicates more precisely the minimum

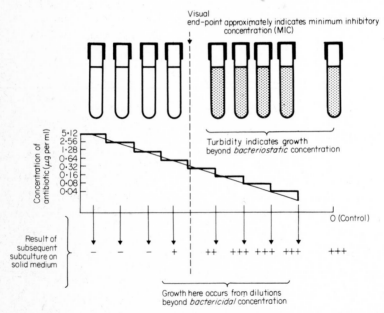

**Figure 13.3** An outline of the determination of bacteriostatic and bactericidal levels of an antibiotic for a given organism.

inhibitory concentration (MIC) of the antibiotic for the test organism and distinguishes between the bacteriostatic concentration, the level at which growth is inhibited, and the bactericidal concentration at which subculture from the test dilution yields no viable organisms.

94

**Table 13.3**  Antibacterial drugs.

| Group | Common example | Comment |
|---|---|---|
| Sulphonamides | Sulphadiazine<br>Sulphadimidine | Bacteriostatic |
| Sulphonamide<br>-trimethoprim | Cotrimoxazole | Can be bactericidal |
| Penicillins | Benzyl penicillin | Bactericidal—given by<br>injection |
| | Phenoxymethyl<br>penicillin | Oral preparation |
| | Methicillin<br>Cloxacillin<br>Flucloxacillin | Penicillins resistant to<br>staphylococcal penicillinase |
| | Ampicillin | 'Broad-spectrum' |
| | Carbenicillin | Useful against *Pseudomonas* |
| Cephalosporins | Cephalothin<br>Cephalexin | Bactericidal; resemble<br>ampicillin in action |
| Aminoglycosides | Streptomycin<br>Kanamycin<br>Gentamicin | Bactericidal, but have<br>toxic effects on nerves<br>of hearing & balance |
| Tetracyclines | Tetracycline<br>Oxytetracycline<br>Chlortetracycline | Bacteriostatic; 'broad-<br>spectrum' effect |
| Chloramphenicol | Chloramphenicol | Bacteriostatic; 'broad-<br>spectrum'; toxic<br>potential for blood-<br>forming tissues |
| Macrolides | Erythromycin | Bacteriostatic; slowly<br>bactericidal. Useful against<br>G+ cocci; non-toxic |
| Lincomycins | Lincomycin<br>Clindamycin | Resemble erythromy-<br>cin in action; also<br>useful against<br>*Bacteroides* |
| Polymyxins | Polymyxin E (Colistin) | Toxic but was useful against<br>*Pseudomonas*; local appli-<br>cation sometimes useful |
| Nitroimidazoles | Metronidazole | Useful against protozoa<br>and anaerobic bacteria |
| Rifamycins | Rifampicin | Bactericidal; of special<br>use in tuberculosis |

# ANTIBACTERIAL AGENTS

## The Sulphonamides

The successful clinical application of the sulphonamide series of drugs exploited the ability of these compounds to compete for the active site of a bacterial enzyme that synthesizes the coenzyme folic acid from $p$-aminobenzoic acid. Human cells must absorb ready-made folic acid, but many bacteria lack the necessary absorption mechanism for this and depend upon intracellular synthesis of the coenzyme.

## Trimethoprim-Sulphonamide: The sequential blockade

A subsequent development took further advantage of this metabolic pathway when it was found that the drug trimethoprim interferes with the action of dihydrofolic acid reductase—an enzyme involved in the pathway that uses the synthesized folate for the biosynthesis of purines and pyrimidines. This is of key importance in nucleic acid synthesis. Man also performs this biosynthesis but, by a happy chance, trimethoprim binds very much more strongly to the bacterial reductase than to the mammalian counterpart. When a sulphonamide drug and a trimethoprim compound are given together in the correct dosage, two sequential links in an essential bacterial chain are thus broken and bacterial growth is stopped (Fig. 13.4). Such a combination has a high *therapeutic index* i.e. it is very usefully toxic to many pathogenic bacteria and relatively non-toxic to man. It is not completely non-toxic in clinical use and there are some people who may react badly; here is an example of the fact that the biological sciences seldom declare such bonuses without reservations that in turn provide evidence of the unity of biochemistry.

## Metronidazole

This is an interesting drug originally developed for its anti-trichomonas activity and of practical use in the treatment of a common protozoal infection of the vagina. It has clinically useful activity against the organisms of Vincent's infection of the mouth in which a spirochaete and one of the *Bacteroides-Fusobacterium* group are involved. The drug is also effective against other anaerobic pathogenic bacteria and may have a wider application in this field.

## The Penicillins

In fact, a weak point in the notion of the unity of biochemistry is that some living things seem to have unique components. A good example is that the cell walls of prokaryotic organisms are braced by a mucopeptide polymer cross-linked by polypeptides; the amino sugars and the polypeptide components include chemicals that are not found in eukaryotic cells (see Vol. 1, p.18). Paradoxically, the synthesis and linking of these materials associated with the physical strength of the bacterial cell wall provides an Achilles' heel that affords opportunities for a very selective antimicrobial strategy; penicillin attacks growing bacteria at this point and kills them. Penicillin inhibits the enzyme glycopeptide transpeptidase concerned in the cross-linking of peptide chains

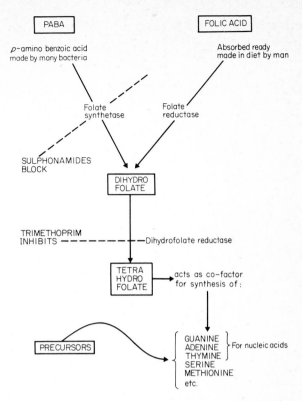

**Figure 13.4**  The sequential blockade produced by the components of co-trimoxazole in the folate pathway.

attached to the glycopeptide (mucopeptide) strands in the cell wall. The structure of penicillin is such that the transpeptidation step is irreversibly blocked. Bacteria affected by penicillin in this way are deprived of the protection of the cell wall and are distorted and disrupted by osmotic forces as they grow.

The drug is essentially non-toxic to man whose cells have a completely different architecture devoid of such corsetry. However, nature has not tolerated this unfair advantage: some bacteria can protect themselves against access of penicillin to their vital framework, and some destroy penicillin by producing potent penicillinases ($\beta$-lactamases); and man has tended to abuse this drug so that some humans have become allergic to it (sensitization).

*Crystalline benzyl penicillin*, the original product and still the best antibiotic of all, is effective against the pathogenic Gram-positive and Gram-negative cocci, and it is also effective against the clostridia, the diphtheria bacillus and the treponema of syphilis. Unfortunately, penicillinase production among the staphylococci severely limits the use of benzyl penicillin against staphylococcal infections and it is generally ineffective against Gram-negative bacilli and mycobacteria. It is not stable in gastric acid and must be given by injection.

More recently developed penicillins include *phenoxymethyl penicillin* which is well absorbed from the alimentary tract and is taken orally; *phenethicillin* and *propicillin* are also acid-resistant and are given orally.

## Penicillinase-resistant penicillins

*Methicillin* is not acid-resistant and must be given by injection, but it is resistant to staphylococcal penicillinase. *Cloxacillin* and *flucloxacillin* are penicillinase-resistant but are also acid-resistant and can be given orally; flucloxacillin is better absorbed. These are regarded as marginally less effective than benzyl penicillin and they only have merit in dealing with penicillinase-producing staphylococci; they are not effective against Gram-negative bacilli.

## 'Broad-spectrum' penicillins

*Ampicillin* is an acid-resistant penicillin with clinically effective activity against a wide range of bacteria including *Escherichia coli, Proteus* spp., *Salmonella* spp. and *Haemophilus influenzae.* It is quite well absorbed from the intestine and is usually given orally; it can also be given by injection. *It is not resistant to penicillinase* and it is often prescribed wrongly for infections caused by penicillinase-producing staphylococci. Ampicillin is also relatively inactive against *Klebsiella* spp. and *Pseudomonas* spp. *Amoxycillin* is a later development from ampicillin and is better absorbed.

Carbenicillin is active against *Pseudomonas aeruginosa.* It must be given by injection.

## The Cephalosporins

This group of antibiotics has activity against a range of organisms including staphylococci, streptococci, neisseriae and coliform bacilli. They act like penicillin on bacterial cell walls and they have been used as alternatives to penicillin for the treatment of infections in patients sensitized to that antibiotic or for the treatment of infections caused by penicillinase-producing staphylococci. In addition, the cephalosporins' clinically useful activity against coliform organisms is sometimes exploited in the special treatment of infection of the urinary tract. The earlier cephalosporin preparations were given by injection; later preparations (cephalexin, cephradine) are given orally.

## Streptomycin

This antibiotic interferes with ribosomal attachment to mRNA and thereby blocks the initiation of protein synthesis. The antibiotic is bactericidal. It is the first of the aminoglycoside group of antibiotics and as it is not absorbed from the gut it is generally given by injection. If a local effect in the intestine is desired, *neomycin* is used—but it is often abused in this respect.

Streptomycin has a wider range of activity than benzyl penicillin and it was the first of the antibiotics to be discovered with effective activity against the tubercle bacillus. Unfortunately, the clinical use of streptomycin is limited by its toxic effects, principally affecting the nerves of hearing and the balancing (vestibular) apparatus in the middle ear; the drug's use is also limited by the rapidity with which bacterial resistance develops to it.

Streptomycin can be valuable in the management of various infections, but its use tends to be largely restricted in view of its very valuable anti-tuberculous activity. It is then used in combination with one or two other antibacterial drugs to counter the development and emergence of resistant bacterial strains (see p.103).

## Gentamicin

This antibiotic is more active against a wider range of organisms than its colleagues in the aminoglycoside group, but it too is toxic for the middle ear. It is bactericidal and is quite widely used for the treatment of *serious* infections caused by coliform bacilli, including so-called 'Gram-negative septicaemia'— especially as it has a useful degree of activity against *Pseudomonas aeruginosa*. The decision to use this drug must be weighed against the knowledge of its toxicity. During treatment with gentamicin, the serum concentrations of the drug are carefully monitored.

## The Tetracyclines

This group of broad-spectrum antibiotics interferes with microbial protein synthesis at the ribosomal level by interfering with the binding of aminoacyl tRNA; it is essentially bacteriostatic for a very wide range of organisms including rickettsiae, chlamydiae and *Mycoplasma pneumoniae*. Tetracyclines are usually given orally and they tend to upset the normal commensal flora. Side-effects include occasional gastro-intestinal upsets. As the tetracyclines are sequestered in growing bone and teeth (which they then stain), their use is not recommended during pregnancy or childhood.

Tetracycline, oxytetracycline and chlortetracycline are all in clinical use and are similar in their activity. These drugs are very widely used, and abused, because of their remarkably broad spectrum and ease of administration. Particularly in the management of respiratory tract infections in general practice, the tetracyclines have been fully exploited in modern medicine. However, it should be noted that the bacteriostatic tetracyclines are not as effective as the properly chosen bactericidal antibiotic in the treatment of certain acute infections, for example in streptococcal disease, and it should be borne in mind that bacterial resistance to the tetracyclines is quite common. Moreover, the tetracyclines may be involved in the increase in transferable drug resistance among bacteria.

## Chloramphenicol

The story of chloramphenicol is the 'hard-luck story' of modern pharmaceutical research. This remarkable antibiotic is purely bacteriostatic; it inhibits protein synthesis by upsetting ribosomal peptidyl transferase in a range of bacteria, rickettsiae and chlamydiae similar to that covered by the tetracyclines, and it is usually given orally. Bacterial resistance normally develops relatively slowly to chloramphenicol, but resistance transfer can occur and this has worrying clinical implications in view of its special place in the treatment of typhoid (see below). In general, the antibiotic is well tolerated and its side-effects are acceptable—except for one dreadful group of problems associated with this antibiotic's occasional effect on the blood-cell-forming tissues in the bone marrow. When this occurs the patient's life is in danger and the condition is sometimes fatally irreversible. Accordingly, the use of this antibiotic is restricted to the treatment of life-threatening conditions in which the risk of the infection outweighs the risk of the treatment. In particular, chloramphenicol is of real clinical use in the treatment of typhoid fever and meningitis caused by *Haemophilus influenzae*.

Chloramphenicol is largely excreted in an inactive form in the urine. This provides a good example of the importance of knowing not only the effect that a drug might have on an organism and the effect of the drug on the patient, but also the effect of the patient's metabolism on the drug.

### Erythromycin

This is one of the macrolide group. It blocks microbial protein synthesis by interfering with the translation stage at the ribosome. It is usually given in oral preparations that protect the base from gastric acid and it is remarkably free from toxic effects or side effects, though erythromycin estolate may cause liver damage. Erythromycin is bacteriostatic, and to some extent bactericidal against Gram-positive cocci and the neisseriae and *Haemophilus influenzae*. It is also active against *Mycoplasma pneumoniae*. Erythromycin is of use in the treatment of penicillin-resistant staphylococcal infections and it has clinically useful activity against streptococci, pneumococci, clostridia and *Bacteroides* species.

### The Lincomycins

Clindamycin (7-chloro lincomycin) the preferred preparation has a spectrum of activity rather like that of erythromycin. It has special merit in the treatment of coccal infections of bone. Its activity against penicillin-resistant staphylococci is useful and it has a particularly effective role in the treatment of infections caused by *Bacteroides* species in clinical practice and in dental practice. The therapeutic use of the lincomycins has been associated with the development of an acute colitis in some patients; there is debate and dispute about this complication which may have been overstated, but the use of this group of antibiotics is likely to be limited until the risk of the complication is defined.

### The Polymyxins

Polymyxin B and Polymyxin E (colistin) are rather toxic antibiotics with clinically useful activity against *Pseudomonas aeruginosa*.

# ANTIFUNGAL THERAPY

**Table 13.4**   Antifungal (antimycotic) drugs.

| Group | Common example | Comment |
|---|---|---|
| (Colchicine-like) | Griseofulvin | Usefully active against ringworm fungi |
| Polyenes | Nystatin | Usefully active against *Candida* (thrush) and some other fungal infections but not ringworm |
|  | Amphotericin B | Useful against some systemic fungal infections, but toxic |

## Griseofulvin and dermatophyte infections

*Griseofulvin* is an antifungal antibiotic produced by a *Penicillium* mould. It is relatively non-toxic, though it may give rise to psychic disturbances in high or cumulative dosage. It is very effective in the systemic treatment of superficial ringworm (dermatophyte) infections which affect the hair, the skin and the nails; the use of this drug has transformed the therapy and the prognosis in many cases. Griseofulvin is not effective against *Candida* infections or the causative agents of the deep (systemic) fungal diseases.

## The Polyene Antibiotics

*Nystatin* and *amphotericin B* both belong to the polyene group of antibiotics used in the treatment of fungal infections. The polyenes seem to combine with sterols in the cytoplasmic membrane and damage it. Sterols do not occur in bacterial cell membranes, hence polyene antibiotics are not antibacterial. However, sterols occur in human cells and man is therefore vulnerable to the cytotoxic effects of polyenes which must be used with care. Nystatin is a useful local agent active against *Candida* but not against the ringworm fungi. Amphotericin B is also active against *Candida* and can be used locally as an alternative if nystatin fails; however, despite its considerably toxicity, the major role of amphotericin B is as a systemic antifungal drug. It is used, with careful monitoring, when a patient is seriously ill with a systemic fungal infection. The drug's continuing and limited role in this field indicates the extent of our requirement for a clinically more acceptable antifungal agent for systemic use against serious infections. 5-fluorocytosine, an alternative to amphotericin B, is unfortunately of the same order of toxicity.

# ANTIVIRAL AGENTS

The pathogenic viruses employ much more subtle mechanisms than do bacteria to upset the host's metabolism and cause disease. It is doubtful whether viruses can be regarded as parasites and, as they essentially redirect host systems to their own ends, the problem of finding an agent with selective toxicity for a viral pathogen, and not for the host cell, is a difficult challenge (see Table 13.5).

**Table 13.5**  Antiviral drugs.

| Group | Example | Comment |
|---|---|---|
| Interferons | Human Interferon | Early promise not yet really fulfilled |
| Pyrimidine analogues: (Thymidine) | 5-iodo-2$'$-Deoxyuridine (Idoxuridine) Trifluorothymidine | Usefully active against Herpes Simplex and Shingles (Herpes Zoster) and vaccinia virus* |
| (Cytidine) | Cytarabine Vidarabine | |
| Thiosemicarbazones | Methisazone | May be of use in prevention of smallpox after exposure to the infection |
| Adamantanes | Amantadine Rimantadine | Have some preventive effect after exposure to influnza (p.103) |
| Dyes | Neutral Red Flavine | Experimental treatment of recurrent herpes |

  * The vaccinia virus used for immunization against smallpox occasionally causes a progressive or generalized infection. In such circumstances, an effective antiviral agent is required.

## Interferon

Cells infected with viruses produce a protein called interferon which inhibits viral attack systems. When human or animal cells are challenged with appropriate viruses *in vitro* or *in vivo*, interferon is produced and this inhibits the multiplication of the challenging virus; it is also inhibitory to other viruses to which the particular cells are normally susceptible. The synthesis of interferon in cells may also be induced by inactivated viruses and by some fungi, bacteria, rickettsiae and chlamydiae. It can also be induced by synthetic double-stranded RNA. The inhibitor is therefore clearly not specific in terms of the inducing agent, but the interferon produced by the cells of one animal species is rather specifically protective for the cells of that species. Accordingly, interferon intended for human use would be most likely to be effective if it is produced by human cells. There is evidence that interferon can prevent the development of the common cold, but the clinical application of interferon is still in the research stage.

## Chemical Antiviral Agents

The following agents are of interest. In general, their toxicity and cost greatly limit their present use. Pyrimidine analogues are usefully active against herpesviruses and vaccinia. They appear to cause miscoding of viral DNA and are not effective against RNA viruses. The thymidine analogue 5-iodo-2'-deoxyuridine (idoxuridine) is used for local application in a dimethyl sulphoxide vehicle to herpes simplex and herpes zoster lesions, especially those involving the eye. *Trifluorothymidine* is also promising. The cytidine analogues *cytarabine* and *vidarabine* are also active against herpes viruses and vaccinia.

The thiosemicarbazone *methisazone* is usefully active against vaccinia virus and is used to treat complications of smallpox vaccination; apparently the drug can be used to moderate the reaction to primary vaccination in an adult, and it is able to interfere with the development of smallpox in unvaccinated persons who have been exposed to the infection. The adamantanes, *amantadine* and *rimantadine* are active against RNA viruses and seem to interfere with the development of certain strains of influenza virus in exposed persons, but the effect is apparently not reliable.

## Local application of dyes

The postulated treatment of certain recurrent herpesvirus infections with one of the dyes is based on the knowledge that certain dyes are adsorbed to the viral nucleic acid. The treated area is then exposed to strong fluorescent light and a 'photodynamic action' is attributed to absorption of damaging energy by the dye with consequent deletions in the viral nucleic acid. Clinical evaluation of this approach is awaited. There are some theoretically worrying hazards.

## ANTIBIOTIC RESISTANCE

The classical mechanism of acquired resistance is the selection by antibiotics of spontaneous mutants that have resistance to increased levels of antibiotics. This can occur *in vivo* or in the environment. A good example of the prompt emergence of strains with marked resistance is found in tuberculosis.

When a case of tuberculosis is diagnosed, the patient already harbours a large number of organisms, and these may include a few spontaneous mutants resistant to any of the commonly used drugs. Treatment with one drug will select for these and the patient will relapse after a few months of therapy, because, in tuberculosis, the normal defence mechanisms cannot mop up the resistant survivors. When we use two or three drugs in combination the mutants resistant to each are killed by the other drugs and we prevent the emergence of resistance. This one-step development and emergence of resistance is particularly associated with streptomycin. The development of resistance *in vivo* and subsequent relapse of the infection is not so commonly encountered in cases of acute infection treated with other antimicrobial drugs, though it can certainly occur—in urinary tract infection for example.

A more common situation, particularly seen in hospital practice, is as follows. When antibiotics are used freely, naturally resistant organisms have a survival advantage and there is an ecological change. As the pyogenic cocci began to be controlled by antimicrobial therapy, the Gram-negative 'coliform' organisms came into prominence as opportunists and are now common causes of wound infection among hospital patients. However, the staphylococci were never really beaten. At the time when penicillin was introduced, a very small proportion of staphylococci were naturally resistant because they produced the enzyme penicillinase which destroys the antibiotic. With the increasing use of penicillin, these strains with the gene carrying the penicillinase information were selected and became relatively more numerous. Unfortunately, the gene can be passed to other staphylococci by a process involving bacterio-phage (transduction); thus, penicillinase-producing staphylococci are now very common, especially in the hospital environment, and simple benzyl penicillin is not likely to control a staphylococcal infection acquired in hospital.

The situation is even more complex. As the staphylococcus persists in the hospital environment, resistance to a wide range of antibiotics is gradually built up by the sequential selection of mutants, each of which might represent only a small increase in degree or range of resistance. There is not typically a single large step in resistance within the population of staphylococci infecting a patient, but there are multiple small steps in the populations of staphylococci that are mixed and exchanged among the personnel and patients in the hospital. From time to time, transduction of resistance information borne on small bits of DNA (plasmids) can occur between staphylococci by phage action.

In the Gram-negative coliforms, transfer of ready-formed resistance genes also occurs. Here the genes are not transferred by bacteriophage, which is a relatively inefficient process. In coliform organisms they are transferred by *conjugation*; this is a sex-like process that allows a much more rapid spread. The resistance genes are contained on R factors, which are bits of DNA that can exist in the cytoplasm of Gram-negative bacilli. These can transfer themselves into other coliform organisms and spread not only to other strains of the same species but also to other species of Gram-negative bacilli. Thus there is a fairly free exchange of R factors between *Escherichia, Salmonella, Shigella* and *Proteus*, and they can even be transferred into more unrelated species such as *Pseudomonas, Vibrio* and *Pasteurella* spp. These groups include many commensals and pathogens for man and animals and in the last 10 years, under the selective pressures of medical, dental, veterinary and other uses of antibiotics, R factors have become widely spread in them. R factors containing as many as 7 or 8 different resistance genes with the ability to confer multiple resistance have been found in Britain in food-poisoning salmonellae and in commensal *Esch. coli* in the gut of patients.

# 14 Preventive microbiology

Control or prevention of infection in a community or family may be considered under three headings (see Fig. 14.1):

A  Eliminate the source or reservoir of infection by early recognition, and effective isolation and treatment of cases and carriers.

B  Define mechanisms of spread of infections and counter these by instruction and engineering.

C  Increase the resistance of the community to infectious diseases, with special reference to those individuals or groups who may be at special risk.

Some of the principles involved in the effective recognition and treatment of infection have been discussed in this book but, in practice, there are many difficulties: Carriers of typhoid and subclinical cases of dysentery are easily missed. Cases of various infections are infectious during the incubation period before the disease is likely to be diagnosed; and the specific treatment of many diseases ranging from the common cold to smallpox is still not possible. For many reasons, prevention is a better and a more practical goal.

The importance of preventive instruction and preventive engineering is readily seen in relation to such diseases as bacillary dysentery, bacterial food poisoning and cholera. In these cases, trouble can be averted by the observation of principles and practices based upon our understanding of the chains of events that lead to the presentation of the dangerous challenges. Once the challenge is allowed to materialize, our therapeutic resources are strained and may fail to cope with the situation. We tend to take for granted safe water supplies, effective sewage disposal systems, clean air, and clean food; but it is clear that, as we increasingly contaminate our environment, increased awareness of the importance of preventive microbiology is called for.

## HOST RESISTANCE TO MICROBIAL INFECTION

Factors that may influence the host-parasite association have already been outlined (pp.31, 34, 42). It is important to note that we are at a disadvantage at the extremes of age; the new-born baby is highly vulnerable to various infective hazards, and old people fare relatively badly for example when flu becomes epidemic. The vulnerability of extreme youth is partly attributable to the immaturity of the immunological and non-specific defences, whereas old age is associated with a great range of degenerative changes that can adversely affect the structure and function of antimicrobial barriers and systems.

It is natural to relate some of our vulnerability to dietary or nutritional deficiencies. Whilst it is true that patients lacking certain vitamins, such as vitamins A and D, vitamin C and vitamins of the B group, may suffer from

**A** *SUPPRESS THE SOURCE*: The prompt detection, isolation and treatment of cases and carriers.

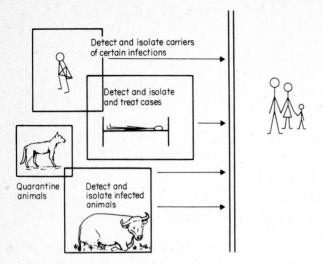

**B** *TACKLE THE TRANSMISSION*: Counter mechanisms of spread by engineering and instruction, e.g. sewage, foodhandling, pasteurization and ventilation.

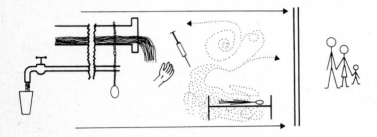

**C** *RAISE HOST RESISTANCE*: Increase resistance by active immunization against specific infections.

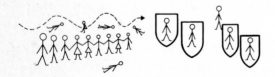

**Figure 14.1**  Approaches to preventive microbiology.

complicating infections, it is quite difficult to prove a direct relationship between susceptibility to infection and subnutrition. On the other hand, various congenital or acquired abnormalities of structure or function, for example in the urinary tract or respiratory tract, are quite clearly associated

106

with an increased susceptibility to infection with a known range of organisms. Furthermore, the relationship of some genetically determined immunological deficiency states with susceptibility to certain infectious agents is readily demonstrable (p.31).

## ACTIVE AND PASSIVE IMMUNIZATION

Specific protection of a potential host against various infections can be conferred by the provision of suitable antibodies in the bloodstream. Antibodies may be antibacterial, or antitoxic, or antiviral, depending upon the antigen that provoked them. If the antibodies are produced in another host and given by injection, or transferred transplacentally in the case of the foetus, the immunity conferred on the recipient is said to be passively acquired or *passive*. The antiserum may be produced in a horse or other animal, or it may be produced in another human being. If the antiserum is refined, fractionated and concentrated, the *gamma globulin fraction* contains the immunoglobulins and these include the protective antibodies (p.27).

The conferring of passive immunity by the injection of antiserum can achieve a prompt concentration of protective antibody in the bloodstream (Fig. 14.2). This is of clinical use in a relative emergency for example to protect

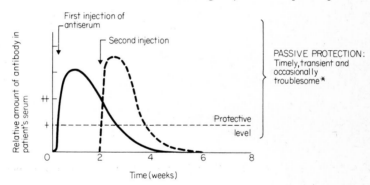

**Figure 14.2** Passive immunity conferred by the injection of antiserum is transient. If the serum is from another species, a second dose tends to be more rapidly eliminated. * Unwelcome side-effects occasionally occur.

a person considered to be at special risk of infection with diphtheria or tetanus or measles etc. However, the level of passively acquired antibody falls quite promptly. Moreover, if an animal serum is used, as is the case with diphtheria antitoxin for example, some people develop severe and potentially dangerous sensitivity reactions to it. The protection is a little less transient and certainly less dangerous if human gamma globulin containing the protective antibody is available.

When antibodies are produced *directly* by the host in response to the administration of an antigen, the immunity is said to be actively acquired or *active*. The production of active immunity takes time and is not generally of use in an emergency. After the first dose of a new antigen, there is a comparatively weak 'priming' response. If the dose is repeated after some weeks, the typical secondary response occurs and a protective level of antibody is then achieved (Fig. 14.3). Thereafter, this can be boosted at suitable intervals

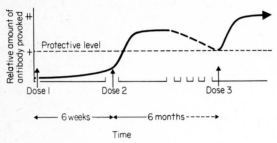

ACTIVE PROTECTION:
Delayed, then durable

**Figure 14.3** Active immunization. The secondary response that follows the administration of a second dose of antigen confers protection. A third (booster) dose provides a durable immunity that may last for years.

depending upon the efficacy of the antigen and various other circumstances. Clinically useful vaccines are generally based on the following antigenic preparations:

(1) *Bacterial toxoid.* This is a bacterial toxin that has been rendered non-toxic by a procedure that retains its effective antigenicity. A toxoid injected under suitable conditions stimulates the production of antibody (antitoxin) that neutralizes the homologous toxin.

(2) *Inactivated ('killed') organisms.* Certain organisms inactivated by selected agents under controlled conditions retain antigenic groups of importance in pathogenicity. The injection of such a preparation under suitable conditions stimulates the production of protective antibodies. Some organisms do not retain their protective antigens when they are treated with inactivating agents.

(3) *Live (attenuated) organisms.* In some cases it has been possible to produce an effective vaccine based on a living strain of an organism that has been treated and selected under conditions whereby its virulence has been fixed at a low level (attenuated). If the strain is not sufficiently attenuated it is dangerous— and if it is unduly attenuated, it is likely to be non-protective or inadequately protective.

Live vaccines in current use include:

 (i) BCG (Bacille Calmette-Guérin) which is an attenuated bovine strain of tubercle bacillus;

 (ii) Oral poliovirus vaccine, which is a mixture of the 3 types of poliovirus in attenuated form;

(iii) Measles vaccine, and

(iv) Rubella vaccine.

## ACTIVE IMMUNIZATION SCHEDULES

During the first few months of life, passively acquired maternal antibodies are

108

gradually lost. At about 6 months (and not earlier than 3 months) it is advisable to begin active immunization against certain diseases, always provided that due account is taken of the following principle enunciated by Professor George Dick: 'Before introducing or retaining any immunization procedure, epidemiological data must be available ... that the disease is of such severity, frequency or other importance as to justify immunization against it.' Side-effects associated with immunization procedures are partly attributable to human errors and partly to inherent deficiencies in certain vaccines. Smallpox vaccination involves an occasional risk of local sepsis and sometimes more serious complications. Whooping-cough vaccine sometimes gives rise to febrile convulsions and occasionally causes cerebral upsets. A serious neurological reaction is a recognized complication of vaccination against rabies. Typhoid-paratyphoid vaccine (T.A.B. vaccine) contains bacterial endotoxin and this may cause a feverish reaction and malaise.

## Schedule

In Britain, the schedule that is presently recommended may be summarized as follows:

Three doses of a vaccine containing diphtheria toxoid, tetanus toxoid and killed *Bordetella pertussis* organisms ('dip-pertussis-tet'; 'triple vaccine') are given at intervals of about 6 weeks and about 6 months to protect the child against diphtheria, whooping cough and tetanus. A dose of oral polio vaccine given on each of these occasions immunizes against poliomyelitis.

A dose of live measles vaccine may be given early in the second year of life.

At school entry age (5 years), a booster dose of diphtheria toxoid and tetanus toxoid given as one shot of a mixed vaccine, and a booster dose of oral polio vaccine are given.

At age 10–13, BCG vaccine is given to tuberculin-negative children, and live rubella vaccine is given to all girls.

At age 15, a further dose of tetanus toxoid covers the accident-prone decade of 15–25, and a further dose of oral polio vaccine is given.

The footnote to the immunization schedule issued in Britain (Table 14.1) contains the following advice:

'In view of the success of the World Health Organization smallpox eradication programme, vaccination against smallpox is no longer recommended as a routine procedure in this country. It is essential, however, that health service staff, including hospital doctors and nurses, public health staff and ambulance workers, who may come in contact with patients, should be adequately vaccinated against smallpox. Doctors, nurses and others on the staff of smallpox hospitals, selected ambulance personnel and others who may have to deal at short notice with smallpox cases, should be revaccinated regularly at not more than yearly intervals. Staff of other hospitals, who may meet unrecognized cases of smallpox or come in contact with infected material from them, public health staff and other ambulance personnel should be offered revaccination at least once every three years. All travellers to areas of the world where smallpox occurs or to countries where eradication programmes are in progress should be protected by recent vaccination.'

**Table 14.1** Schedule of vaccination and immunization procedures—1972—extracted with

| Age | Vaccine |
| --- | --- |
| During the first year of life. | Diphtheria/Tetanus/Pertussis and oral polio vaccine (First dose) |
| | Diphtheria/Tetanus/Pertussis and oral polio vaccine (Second dose) |
| | Diphtheria/Tetanus/Pertussis and oral polio vaccine (Third dose) |
| During the second year of life. | Measles vaccine. |
| At 5 years of age or school entry. | Diphtheria/Tetanus and oral polio vaccine or Diphtheria/Tetanus/Polio vaccine. |
| Between 10 and 13 years of age. | BCG vaccine. |
| All girls aged 11 to 13 years. | Rubella vaccine. |
| At 15 to 19 years of age or on leaving school. | Polio vaccine (oral or inactivated) and tetanus toxoid. |

Whilst this British schedule may serve as a useful guide, it is most important that a schedule followed in another country must take account of the local infectious hazards and priorities of that country. Moreover, any immunization schedule must take account of the resources of finance, organization and skilled personnel required for its implementation and its maintenance.

This statement illustrates the difficulties that arise when the stage of partial success is reached in an eradication programme coupled with the extension of a vaccination policy that involves the use of an imperfect vaccine against a dangerous disease of fairly high infectivity.

| Interval | Notes |
|---|---|
| Preferably after an interval of 6 to 8 weeks.<br><br>Preferably after an interval of 4 to 6 months. | The earliest age at which the first dose should be given is 3 months, but a better general immunological response can be expected if the first dose is delayed to 6 months of age. |
| After an interval of not less than 3 weeks. | Although measles vaccination can be given in the second year of life, delay until the age of three years or more will reduce the risk of occasional severe reactions to the vaccine. |
|  | These may be given, if desired, at 3 years of age to children entering nursery schools, attending day nurseries or living in children's homes. |
|  | For tuberculin-negative children. |
| There should be an interval of not less than 3 weeks between BCG and rubella vaccination. | All girls of this age should be offered rubella vaccine whether or not there is a past history of an attack of rubella. |

## SAFETY IN THE LABORATORY

The first principle is that no micro-organism can be said to be harmless to man. There is a potential risk in handling any organism; this ranges from the obvious hazard of a known pathogen, to the often overlooked risk of sensitization to the most benign. This small book has failed if the reader is not now convinced that circumstances that might lead to disease are endlessly variable and that organisms can evolve infinitely to take advantage of changes in man's external and internal environment.

Fundamental safety rules in the microbiological laboratory are based on the concepts of sources and transmission of infection that have been outlined. It is particularly important to relate these to a qualitative appreciation of the relative virulence of various recognized pathogens and to a quantitative appreciation of challenge doses (p.32) that can be delivered by various routes. It is clearly essential to observe the following general rules and to understand that many others must be formulated for specific situations:

Eating, drinking, smoking, the licking of labels and the use of pipettes by mouth are forbidden in a microbiological laboratory. Food or drink destined for consumption must not be stored in a laboratory refrigerator.

Dangerous aerosols may be produced when a container holding a microbial suspension is opened, or when the suspension is poured or mixed or pipetted. Aerosols are particularly likely to be produced during homogenization procedures or when syringes, pumps and centrifuges are used.

Accidental inoculation is a constant risk—usually associated with laboratory breakages but less obviously occurring, for example, when splintered woodwork is contaminated. Straight wires and needles must be handled with additional care when they are charged with organisms. Drawing pins, compasses and dividers and other sharp or pointed instruments should be kept away from the bacteriological bench unless there is a special requirement for them there. *Injuries regularly occur when inexperienced workers attempt to push glass tubing into rigid rubber or plastic connections.*

A microbiological laboratory should be 'uncluttered'. Its organization and good management should be evident; otherwise there is a real risk of cross-infection of personnel, including cleaning staff, and cross-contamination of experiments. The disposal of all cultures and contaminated materials must be rigidly controlled and an absolutely dependable disinfection or sterilization procedure must be included. This applies to disposable and non-disposable items, which should be dealt with separately. The proper disposal of contaminated broken glass demands special care and consideration for others.

# Suggestions for further reading

**Chapters 1 and 2**  General texts on medical microbiology

CRUICKSHANK R., DUGUID J.P., MARMION B.P. and SWAIN R.H.A. (editors) (1973) *Medical Microbiology*. Churchill-Livingstone, Edinburgh & London.
Volume 1 contains a wealth of information on infectious agents, infection and immunity.

GILLIES R.R. (1975) *Lecture Notes on Medical Microbiology* (2nd edition). Blackwell Scientific Publications, Oxford, London, Edinburgh & Melbourne.
A clear and concise account.

DAVIS B.D., DULBECCO R., EISEN H.N., GINSBERG H.S. and WOOD B. (1968) *Microbiology*. Harper & Row, New York, Evanston & London.
This is a fine text with many good illustrations.

PASSMORE R. and ROBSON J.S. (editors) (1973) *A Companion to Medical Studies*. Volume 2, revised reprint. Blackwell Scientific Publications, Oxford, London, Edinburgh & Melbourne.
This volume deals with Pharmacology, Microbiology, General Pathology and related subjects.

**Chapter 3**

TIMBURY M.C. (1974) *Notes on Medical Virology* (5th edition). Churchill-Livingstone, Edinburgh & London.
A lucid summary and a useful aid for students.

FENNER F., McAUSLAN B.R., MIMS C.A., SAMBROOK J. and WHITE D.O. (1974) *The Biology of Animal Viruses*. Academic Press, New York & London.
This is an authoritative text.

PRIMROSE S.B. (1974) *Introduction to Modern Virology*. Blackwell Scientific Publications, Oxford, London, Edinburgh & Melbourne.
A stimulating introduction to biochemical and genetic aspects of virology.

**Chapter 4**

RIPPON J.W. (1973) Medical Mycology: The Pathogenic Fungi and the Pathogenic Actinomycetes, in *Textbook of Microbiology* (20th edition) edited by W. Burrows. W.B. Saunders Company, Philadelphia, London & Toronto.
This illustrates the breadth of the field and gives many references.

**Chapter 5**

WEIR D.M. (1974) *Immunology for Undergraduates*. Churchill-Livingstone, Edinburgh & London.
A very helpful introduction.

THOMPSON R.A. (1974) *The Practice of Clinical Immunology*. Edward Arnold, London.
This is a clear account of theory and practice.

**Chapter 6**     See the general texts listed above, and note also:

SMITH H. and PEARCE J.H. (editors) (1972) *Microbial Pathogenicity in Man and Animals* (22nd Symposium of the Society for General Microbiology). Cambridge University Press.
This is full of information and ideas.

AJL S.J., CIEGLER A., KADIS S., MONTIE T.C. and WEINBAUM G. (1970-1972) *Microbial Toxins* (Volumes I—VIII). Academic Press, New York & London.
Volumes I—III are devoted to bacterial protein toxins; IV and V to endotoxins; and VI—VIII to fungal and algal toxins. There is much detailed and authoritative information.

**Chapters 7—11**     See the general texts, and note the following:

HOBBS B.C. (1968) *Food Poisoning and Food Hygiene* (2nd edition). Edward Arnold, London.
A basic primer.

RIEMANN H. (editor) (1969) *Food-borne Infections and Intoxications.* Academic Press, New York & London.
An extensive account.

CHRISTIE A.B. (1974) *Infectious Diseases: Epidemiology and Clinical Practice* (2nd edition). Churchill-Livingstone, Edinburgh, London & New York.
This is already a classic and a standard reference.

PASSMORE R. and ROBSON J.S. (editors) (1974) *A Companion to Medical Studies* Volume 3. Blackwell Scientific Publications, Oxford, London, Edinburgh & Melbourne.
Volume 3 is a general medical text with many useful accounts of infections and of communicable diseases.

**Chapter 10**

VERNON E. and TILLETT H.E. (1974) Food poisoning and salmonella infections in England and Wales 1969—1972. *Public Health, London.* **88**, 225.

COLLEE J.G. (1974) Bacterial challenges in food. *Postgraduate Medical Journal.* **50**, 636—43 (With acknowledgement to the Editor for kind permission to reproduce material originally published in this journal).

**Chapter 12**

SYKES G. (1972) *Disinfection and Sterilization* (reprint of revised 2nd edition). Chapman & Hall Ltd., London.
A remarkably comprehensive and authoritative reference work.

RUBBO S.D. and GARDNER J.F. (1965) *A Review of Sterilization and Disinfection.* Lloyd-Luke, London.
This is a very useful book.

KELSEY J.C. and MAURER I.M. (1972) *The Use of Chemical Disinfectants in Hospitals* (PHLS Monograph Series, No. 2). HMSO, London.
This should be required reading for all concerned.

MAURER I.M. (1974) *Hospital Hygiene.* Edward Arnold, London.
Provides answers to practical questions.

**Chapter 13**

GARROD L.P., LAMBERT H.P. and O'GRADY F. (1973) *Antibiotic and Chemotherapy* (4th edition). Churchill-Livingstone, Edinburgh & London.
Comprehensive, authoritative and highly recommended.


**Chapter 14** See the general texts and note also:

COLLINS C.H., HARTLEY E.G. and PILSWORTH R. (1974) *The Prevention of Laboratory Acquired Infection.* (PHLS Monograph Series, No. 6). HMSO London.
Required reading for all who handle potential pathogens.

LOWBURY E.J.L., AYLIFFE G.A.J., GEDDES A.M. and WILLIAMS J.O. (1975) *Control of Hospital Infection: A Practical Handbook.* Chapman & Hall, London.

SHAPTON D.A. and BOARD R.G. (editors) (1972) *Safety in Microbiology* (Soc. appl. Bact. Tech. Series No. 6). Academic Press, London & New York.
This gives helpful practical details.

CENTRAL PATHOLOGY COMMITTEE (1972) *Safety in Pathology Laboratories.* Department of Health & Social Security & Welsh Office, HMSO, London & Edinburgh.
A basic guide to safety measures.

GIBSON G.L. (editor) (1974) *Infection in Hospital* (2nd edition). Churchill-Livingstone, Edinburgh, London & New York.
A useful code of practice.

# Postscript

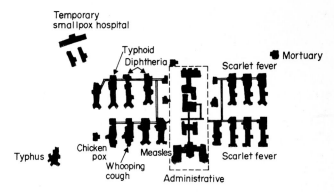

**Figure P** An outline of the lay-out of Edinburgh City Hospital for Infectious Diseases (from a Post Office plan of Edinburgh 1914—15, with acknowledgement to Dr. Stewart Semple). A reminder of significant microbial challenges 60 years ago when our preventive and therapeutic resources were more limited.

# Index

Fever, enteric, 67
rheumatic, 44, 49
scarlet, 44
typhoid, 67
Filamentous bacteria, 1, 4
Filtration, 89
Fixed macrophages, 26
Flagellar H antibodies, 27
Flocculation, 12
Flucloxacillin, 98
Follicular tonsillitis, 49
Fomites, 34
Food poisoning, 71
*Clostridium welchii*, 77
infection type, 72
staphylococcal, 76
toxic types, 76
Fungal, Disease, 21
Fungal, disease, laboratory diagnosis of, 23
hyphae, 24, 25
toxins, 23
Fungi, (including yeasts), 2
dermatophytes, 22
laboratory culture of, 24
pathogenic, 21
Fungus, dimorphic, 21

Gamma rays, 90
Gamma-globulins, 27, 28, 107
Genital herpes, 56
Genome, viral, 17
Gentamicin, 99
Geophilic fungi, 22
Giant cells, 29
Glomerulonephritis, acute, 49
Glutaraldehyde, 88
Gonococcal pus, 53
Gonococcus, 43
Griseofulvin, 101
Guarnieri bodies, 16
Gut, bacterial challenges in, 69

Haemadsorption, 20
Haemagglutination, 14, 20
Haemagglutination-inhibition, 20
Haematogenous, 38
β-Haemolytic streptococcus, 44, 49
*Haemophilus influenzae*, 55, 64
Hand-to-mouth infection, 65
Healthy carrier, 33
Heat-treatment temperatures, 90
Hepatitis, serum, 56 ·
viral, 68
Hepatitis B, viral, 56
Herpes simplex virus, 56
Herpesvirus hominis, 56
Herpesviruses, 19, 56
Hexachlorophane, 86
Hide porter's disease, 79
*Histoplasma capsulatum*, 21
Host, compromised, 43
defence systems, 26
resistance, 105
Host-parasite association, 3, 32
Hot air oven, 89
Humoral, antibodies, 27
immunity, 27

Hyaluronidase, 40
Hyperplasia, 18
Hyphae, fungal, 24, 25
Hypogammaglobulinaemia, 31

ID50, 32
IgA, 27
IgD, 28
IgE, 27
IgG, 27
IgM, 27
Immune response, 26
Immunity, 26
cell-mediated, 27
humoral, 27
passive, 107
Immunization, active, 10, 108
passive, 107
procedures, schedules of, 110
Immunofluorescence procedures, 14
Immunoglobulins, 27, 107
Inapparent infection, 10
Inclusion bodies, 16
Infected dust, 59
Infection, acute toxic, 44
by contact, 35
by ingestion, 35
by inhalation, 35
by inoculation, 35
endogenous, 34
exogenous, 34
exotic, 42
hand-to-mouth, 65
inapparent, 10
latent, 56
opportunistic, 42
respiratory route of, 59
shigella, 65
sub-clinical, 10
type of food poisoning, 72
urinary tract, 53, 54
Infectivity, 32, 37
Inflammation, acute, 28
Influenza virus, 64
Ingestion, infection by, 35
Inhalation, infection by, 35
Inhibition tests, 14
Inoculation, infection by, 35
in clinical practice, 36
Interferon, 102
Intracytoplasmic inclusions, 16
Intradermal, 36
Intraleucocytic, digestion, 30
killing, 30
Intramuscular, 36
Intranuclear inclusions, 16
Intravenous, 36
Invasiveness, 37
5-Iodo-2′-deoxyuridine, 102, 103
Ionizing radiations, 90
Irradiation, ultra-violet, 90
Isopropyl alcohol, 85, 86, 87

Koch-Henle postulates, 8